JUN   2006

W9-CZW-195

HELP YOUR TEENAGER BEAT AN EATING DISORDER

HELP YOUR TEENAGER BEAT AN EATING DISORDER

JAMES LOCK   DANIEL LE GRANGE

THE GUILFORD PRESS
New York   London

© 2005 The Guilford Press
A Division of Guilford Publications, Inc.
72 Spring Street, New York, NY 10012
www.guilford.com

Printed in the United States of America

This book is printed on acid-free paper.

Last digit is print number: 9 8 7 6 5 4 3 2 1

Library of Congress Cataloging-in-Publication Data
Lock, James.
  Help your teenager beat an eating disorder / James Lock, Daniel Le Grange.
    p. cm.
  Includes bibliographical references and index.
  ISBN 1-57230-908-3 (pbk.: alk. paper)—ISBN 1-59385-101-4 (hard cover: alk. paper)
  1. Eating disorders in adolescence—Popular works. 2. Parent and teenager. I. Le Grange, Daniel. II. Title.
  RJ506.E18L63 2005
  616.85′26′00835—dc22
                                                            2004016664

To my children
−JDL

To my mother and late father
−DLG

*We would like to thank all the many patients
and families we have worked with over the years
for helping us learn how best to help them.*

CONTENTS

INTRODUCTION

When your children are sick, you don't just bring them home from the doctor's office or hospital and leave them to their own defenses. If it's the flu, the child needs fluids and rest and medicine to bring the fever down. If it's an allergy, someone needs to check package labels to make sure the allergen isn't included in a food. If your child has asthma, you make sure the inhaler is available and watch vigilantly for signs of an attack. And if your child has a very serious illness, like cancer or heart disease, you don't just expect it to get better on its own.

Someone needs to be there when the doctor isn't. That person is you. Parents are an integral part of the treatment of their children for every illness you can think of. Why, then, should it be different for eating disorders?

It shouldn't. Anorexia nervosa and bulimia nervosa are extremely serious illnesses that can threaten your child's very survival. By their nature, they are self-perpetuating and insidious. That's why a significant proportion of teenagers and adults who have eating disorders end up in the hospital at some point during the course of their illness: They need the constant, consistent vigilance of a team of professionals to ensure that they return to normal weight and normal eating habits.

The trouble is what happens when they get home. Many treatment programs for anorexia and bulimia still advocate keeping parents out of their teenager's care, for a variety of reasons that we explain in this book. The consequence is often a relapse. When an eating disorder still has a hold on a teenager, leaving the child to manage it on her own once she's at home just gives the eating disorder a chance to slip through the flimsy defenses of self-care and send her on a downward spiral toward physical and psychological damage once more.

For more than a decade we have watched adolescents and their parents struggle with this horrible cycle of getting better and then getting worse again. Most of those who come to our offices arrive feeling anxious about their child's bewildering condition and overwhelmed or even defeated by this strange illness. Numerous parents have already been told by other professionals to stay on the sidelines or they will "make things worse." Many are confused in general, not quite knowing whether their child really has an eating disorder, or what precisely an eating disorder is, or what they should do about it.

We wrote this book to clear up misconceptions that we have found—and that the research is beginning to reveal—only make it harder for adolescents to recover from anorexia nervosa, bulimia nervosa, and their variations: that you are to blame for the problem, that your child needs to be treated without any input or involvement (aka "interference") by you, that you need to leave diagnosis and treatment to the professionals in a way you would never agree to if your child had cancer or a heart problem, or even a broken bone. This book therefore has one simple purpose: to help you understand eating disorders and their insidious nature and to show you how you can help your child in "plugging those tiny cracks" where the eating disorder keeps slipping into her or his life.

That doesn't mean this book is a "self-help" manual. Eating disorders are very serious illnesses, and we have no evidence that self-help approaches are sufficient by themselves for adolescents and their families. Instead, this book is intended to provide straight answers and hard facts about eating disorders based on the available research evidence and our own extensive clinical experience. Its goal is to offer you a perspective that is only beginning to emerge: that you have an important role to play in helping your child recover. We believe, in fact, that you are key to your teenager's return to health. This applies whether you are just considering having your child evaluated by a doctor or your child has undergone several other treatments in the past and has not yet conquered this illness. You are certainly in the best possible position to take action fast, before an eating disorder has an opportunity to do serious damage to your child's health. The research shows that when anorexia and bulimia are treated early, there is a good chance of full recovery. So, if nothing else, we hope this book moves you to take your child's problem seriously and get help *now*. Ideally, the book will help you go further than that, however. It should help you establish a foundation on which you and the clinicians you work with can build a successful partnership in defeating the disorder that has overtaken your child. We hope to demystify anorexia and bulimia, and at the same time encourage you to consider how you can help with the problems that such an illness is causing for your child and family.

The parents who come to our offices usually arrive believing they *shouldn't* be involved in helping with their child's eating disorder. This message typically comes from an external source, because few parents would subscribe instinctively to "staying out of it" if their child had any other life-threatening illness. Therefore, this book may appear at first to be taking a radical stance. We hope you'll realize that is not the case when you read the data in Chapter 6 and elsewhere, which show that parents' participation in treatment can make an enormous positive contribution to the recovery of an adolescent with anorexia or bulimia. Regardless of the cause or treatment type, we will argue in this book that you not only can but should be involved. This book will help you figure out how.

The approach we use in our own treatment delivery—one of us currently at Stanford University and the other at the University of Chicago—is derived in concept from decades of family work for anorexia nervosa at the Maudsley Hospital in London. This work illustrates the importance of parents' involvement and support in finding solutions to the dilemmas faced by their adolescents with eating disorders. This perspective stands in stark contrast to approaches that blame parents and exclude them from treatment.

The fact that this book is for parents in the first place sets it apart from most books on eating disorders. Most of these books in print are directed at adults or teenagers themselves who are ill, which has left a big gap in sources of information for parents. That's why we've crafted this book to answer the questions that parents have brought to us over many years of practice—everything from "Am I to blame?" to "What do I do when he disappears after a meal and I know he is going to throw it all up?" "Just how do we get her to eat a healthy meal again when she won't let us?" "Shouldn't she be on some medication as well?" and "I don't understand this illness; isn't the solution straightforward—you eat, and that's that?"

We have been gathering answers to these questions, separately and together, for a combined total of more than 25 years as clinician-researchers (meaning that we see patients and we also conduct research studies) treating adolescents with eating disorders at academic medical centers. Eating disorders are relatively rare, yet each of us has seen hundreds of patients and their parents during this time. We have treated patients in inpatient settings, group programs, and individual and family therapies. We have spent our academic careers exploring how better to help adolescents with eating disorders, and this book is an important part of that effort.

A particular issue that has struck us in a very meaningful way is just how resourceful parents usually are and what a great resource they are when they are brought into the treatment process. We very strongly believe that if parents can be helped to better understand eating disorders and to get involved in taking definite early steps to intervene in these problems in a constructive way, many lives will be improved and some lives actually saved.

Both of us have worked as clinicians and researchers in academic medical settings for the past decade or so. Although we have worked in different parts of the world, our mutual interest in the treatment of adolescents with eating disorders has brought us together in our thinking about how best to do what we do on a daily basis in our respective practices. This has led to a rich and productive collaboration that started in 1998 when we jointly wrote our first book, a manual for clinicians who treat adolescents with anorexia. Since then we have conducted workshops about this treatment throughout the world. We discuss our difficult cases with each other, we present our research findings at professional meetings, and we continue to collaborate on ongoing and new clinical treatment studies. Throughout all this work with adolescents and their parents, we are reminded every day of the real value of parents' contributions to the treatment process. It is this collective experience of treating teenagers with eating disorders, engaging their parents in this process, and researching and writing about these experiences in academic journals that has inspired us to involve parents in the process through writing this book.

HOW TO USE THIS BOOK

This book is divided into three parts. The titles for the chapters were chosen carefully to draw your attention to the urgency of the matter, to highlight the most salient aspects of eating disorders, and then, with this knowledge, to help you respond to your child's illness in the best possible way. If our use of imperatives like "Act Now," "Get Together," and "Don't Waste Time" seems aggressive, it's intended to get your attention. It's human nature to hope that a health problem will go away on its own, but to postpone seeking help for your son or daughter can be extremely dangerous. Sadly, treatment approaches that rob you of your rightful role as guardian of your child's health only encourage you to let others make critical decisions about what to do and when.

In Part I of this book, we focus on *why* you need to take action now if your child has symptoms of an eating disorder. We discuss why eating disorders are serious problems, why you must act together as parents to get treatment started and worry less about "why" this problem developed and more about "how" to get it eradicated. Dealing with eating disorders effectively always requires you to perceive your child's anorexia or bulimia as an urgent matter that needs your prompt attention. In fact, "urgent" is the byword for Part I of this book. It's worth repeating what we said earlier: If your child has signs of an eating disorder, it's urgent that she or he get help, and it's you, the parents, who are in the best possible position to see that your child gets this help.

Part II provides you with more "nuts and bolts" about eating disorders. Eating disorders can be very confusing to doctors, parents, and sufferers alike. Therefore, it's important for you to know what you're up against, perhaps more so than with many other types of illness. The purpose of this section of the book is to make sure you appreciate the complexities of these illnesses. We discuss the various types of eating disorders, particularly anorexia nervosa and bulimia nervosa, as well as how starvation and binge eating and purging can lead to severe medical problems. You will find that we often discuss eating disorders as if they were entities independent of your child. We do this to stress our view that eating disorders are illnesses and not willful choices being made by your child in order to oppose you. Next we illustrate how a teenager with an eating disorder thinks. The distortions common to such thought processes are illustrated to underscore the need for treatment. They can also help you separate the illness from the child so that you can remain supportive of your son or daughter, who is, after all, suffering from real distortions in how he or she experiences his or her body, and in his or her thoughts and beliefs about food and weight. We end this section with information about the main treatment approaches for eating disorders and the evidence available for their effectiveness so that you'll have a good scientific understanding of what may help your child and what may not.

Part III of this book is designed to help you tackle the practical problems you will face in trying to get and use help for your child's eating disorder. We illustrate various ways that parents can be involved in each of the known major treatments for eating disorders, even if the form of treatment discourages parental involvement. We also offer tips to help you confront the cultural forces that contribute to disordered thinking about food and weight. Most important, though, is the partnership that we mentioned earlier. To seal up those cracks that your child's eating disorder will do its best to slip through, the entire treatment team needs to establish a united front to fight the illness. This means that both parents—or you and any other adults who are invested in helping your child recover—need to be "on the same page" in dealing with the illness at all times. It means that you also need to find a way to form a fruitful alliance with the professionals on your treatment team. So this section includes chapters that help you stave off the eating disorder's efforts to "divide and conquer" and help you stand your ground constructively when you have disagreements with the experts who are trying to cure your teenage son or daughter.

WHAT YOU WILL LEARN FROM THIS BOOK

After you have read this book, we hope you will feel confident that you have a role in helping your adolescent in his or her recovery from an eating disorder. You should know the ways in which eating disorders develop and when to get worried as normal adolescents' concerns with their bodies become more serious. You will know the medical problems that can and will develop if your child's eating disorder isn't treated effectively. You will know what to expect when you have your child evaluated and what kinds of treatments are likely to be offered. You will learn that parental involvement can take many forms, such as actually helping your starved child to eat at home, supporting individual therapy for your child, monitoring binge eating and purging episodes, and participating in treatments that enhance your adolescent's interpersonal capacities and roles.

We also hope that after reading this book you will be certain that there is help for your adolescent with an eating disorder and that the resources we provide at the conclusion will be helpful to you in determining where to go for this assistance.

A NOTE FROM THE AUTHORS

This book is not intended as a self-help guide nor is it intended in any way to substitute for the advice of a physician or therapist. Moreover, research into eating disorders, their causes, and the best treatments is ongoing; to stay abreast of advances in the field, consult reliable sources such as those listed in the Resources and Further Reading sections at the end of the book.

This book is aimed at helping parents with older children and adolescents, not young children or adult children.

Eating disorders increasingly affect teenage boys as well as teenage girls, though they are still more common in girls. All statements in this book, unless otherwise noted, apply to both adolescent boys and adolescent girls. To emphasize this point, we alternate pronouns in examples throughout the text.

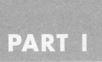

PART I

Getting Started

FIRST STEPS TOWARD HELPING YOUR CHILD
WITH AN EATING DISORDER

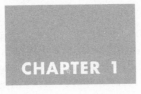

CHAPTER 1

ACT NOW

You don't know what to do.

Thirteen-year-old Sheila has been losing weight for 6 months. At first you thought it was normal teenage dieting. But she's too thin now. She has stopped eating with you but insists on cooking everything for the whole household. Last week she made four desserts but wouldn't eat any of them. She has a book with a list of the calories in everything most of us eat, but she doesn't need it anymore because she knows it by heart. Besides, at present, she eats only three things: raw vegetables, tofu, and dry cereal. She's still doing well in school. Her straight As, though, seem more of a burden than a source of accomplishment to her. When she isn't studying, she's going for a run or doing sit-ups. She ignores calls from her friends and seems more and more depressed. When you try to encourage her to eat, she fumes and says it's none of your business. She insists she's fine.

You don't know what to do.

You caught 17-year-old Donna throwing up. She said she was sick. But it wasn't the first time. You have heard her before.

Always heading off to the bathroom after every meal. She says it was nothing, she only had an upset stomach. You've noticed she hardly eats breakfast or lunch, but when you come home in the evening, lots of food is gone from the pantry, especially cookies, potato chips, and bread. You've had to go to the store midweek to restock. One of her friends told you she was worried about Donna. You are too.

You don't know what to do.

Tom used to be a great high school diver. He's too weak now to perform his toughest dives. He eats only protein bars and fruit drinks. He is constantly exercising to get perfect abdominal muscles, but you can see his ribs. He says he's still too fat. Where there used to be muscle, there's mostly bone and skin now. At first his coach complimented Tom on his weight loss because it had improved his dive entries. Now the coach has called you and suggested Tom take a leave from the team. Tom's best friend called him "skeleton" to tease him, but you know he's worried too.

You don't know what to do. *Should* you do something?

This is the first problem you face if you're concerned that your son or daughter may have an eating disorder. You know most eating problems in children are transient. You remember lots of struggles over junk food and sweets with your other children, or you've seen it in other families. Many children commonly go through periods of being picky eaters, eating more than usual, eating less than usual, and even complaining about upset stomachs or having periods of mild digestive problems and constipation. You've asked other parents and relatives about these types of behaviors and learned that, although usually short-lived, eating problems are nearly universal. As children enter puberty, many, especially girls, are very much interested in their appearance and weight and may try dieting or other weight loss strategies. You expect this because you know it's normal to become more concerned about appearance in the teenage years and because you've known your son's or daughter's friends to express similar thoughts and engage in the same types of behavior. You don't want to create a problem where there isn't one.

How do you know if there's a real problem?

If you think your child's thoughts and behaviors resemble those of Sheila, Donna, or Tom, however, it's time to take action to help. Left untreated, eating disorders can lead to chronic health problems, depression, and even death. With the severe weight loss associated with anorexia nervosa, for example, starvation leads to lower body temperatures, decreased blood pressure, and decreased heart rate, as well as rough and dry skin, loss of hair, loss of menstruation in young women, and osteoporosis. Because the body isn't being fed, it turns to muscle for fuel. This causes weakness, fatigue, and, in particular, decreased cardiac mass (the heart being a large muscle in the body), which can prompt dangerous changes in heart rhythm and may thereby cause cardiac failure and death. Over time, the risk of death as a result of the complications of anorexia is estimated at 6–15%. This mortality rate is the highest for any psychiatric disease.

For bulimia nervosa, the risk for death appears to be lower, but there still are risks of severe medical complications. One of the most common of these is depletion of potassium (hypokalemia), which results from loss of body stores of this essential electrolyte due to purging stomach contents. Without potassium, which is required for many basic physical processes, but significantly important for muscle contraction, cardiac arrhythmias are possible, leading to cardiac arrest and death. In addition, with chronic vomiting, the linings of the esophagus and stomach can become eroded, and this can cause bleeding, ulcers, and even death if the bleeding cannot be stopped. Chronic use of laxatives and purgatives leads to intestinal problems, including pain and severe and unremitting constipation. Both vomiting and the use of laxatives lead to severe depletion of water from the body (dehydration), which can cause low and changing blood pressure, increasing the likelihood of fainting and falls.

We discuss these complications in more detail in Chapter 4. By now, though, you can undoubtedly see that eating disorders have serious health consequences. To be complacent in the face of a possible eating disorder is the greatest risk a parent can take in the battle to prevent such serious problems from developing.

WHAT DOES AN EATING DISORDER LOOK LIKE AS IT DEVELOPS?

If you're to catch a problem before it becomes an eating disorder, you have to know what to look for over time. Sheila, Donna, and Tom's problems did not develop in a day. Like most eating disorders, their problems developed gradually and sometimes in secret. If you understand the path by which more typical, temporary eating problems and weight concerns can become real eating disorders, you can get a sense of where your own child is on that trajectory.

Extreme Dieting: The Path to Anorexia Nervosa

Fourteen-year-old Sydney has always been a terrific child. Her parents said she had spoiled them because she was always so easy, independent, reliable, and mature. That's why they were so shocked by her recent weight loss. She had never shown the slightest sign of emotional problems. She was an honor student, swim team champ, and popular at school. She had never been overweight; in fact, she'd always been on the thin side.

The problems seemed to begin during the summer before ninth grade. Sydney had been on the summer swim team. It was the first time her parents noticed that she wanted to stay longer to swim after practice. She wanted to get fitter, she said, so she could be a starter on both the breaststroke and freestyle teams. At the same time, she started a vegetarian diet. She felt it was cruel to eat animals, and besides, she didn't need fat in her diet when she was trying to be healthier. At first her parents understood and supported her efforts at self-improvement as Sydney seemed happy and confident.

Then Sydney attended the special 3-week swim camp for the summer team located in another part of the state. She left in the middle of July and returned at the end of the first week of August. When her parents picked her up at the bus, they were startled, almost frightened by how thin Sydney had become. They didn't say anything right away. They were just glad to have their daughter home. They surmised that the food hadn't been too good at the camp, and Sydney implied as much. They didn't have good vegetarian choices, she said, and she was very active. She had made both teams as a starter.

And then school began. The ninth grade was a transitional year for Sydney. Students from three middle schools were combined in a single high school, so there were many new kids in her class. Her parents noticed that Sydney seemed more preoccupied and worried about schoolwork, but they thought this was to be expected when starting high school. Sydney's day began at 5:00 A.M. with swim practice for 2 hours before school. She then attended classes for the day and reported for another swim practice from 5:00 to 7:00 P.M. Sydney arrived home after the family had already eaten. She studied until 11:00 P.M.

Out of sight of her parents, Sydney had developed a highly limited eating pattern. She allowed herself one cup of orange juice before morning practice. She told her mother she had a bagel and cream cheese at school with milk after practice, but in reality, she ate half a dry bagel and water. The lunch her mother carefully prepared for her was thrown away each day. Again before afternoon practice, she would drink a glass of orange juice. Because she came home after the family had eaten, her parents didn't know how much she had for dinner. Usually she had a carefully weighed slice of tofu, a few carrots, and an apple.

Her parents grew increasingly alarmed at Sydney's continued weight loss. The coach of the swim team called to ask what was wrong with Sydney. She was afraid that Sydney might have an eating disorder. Her parents made an appointment with her pediatrician, which took some time to set up. When they arrived, the pediatrician said that Sydney was too thin, and Sydney promised to eat more. Unfortu-

nately, she did not. Her parents tried to intervene, but she
became angry easily when they talked to her about eating,
and they hated to confront her.

Although anorexia nervosa usually starts in early adolescence,
typically at 13–14 years, it is not uncommon to see children
between the ages of 8 and 11 develop this eating disorder.
Anorexia usually begins with an episode of dieting that gradually
leads to life-threatening starvation. At times some identifiable
precipitating event triggers the dieting process. Maybe the child
is teased about her weight, or her friends start dieting. Or perhaps she sees her parents dieting. Some girls start dieting at the
onset of menses, when they make the transition to a new school
or level in school, or when they begin dating. The illness of a parent may also trigger dieting. It's important to understand that
these events often start the dieting process, but that does not
mean these triggers are the causes of anorexia nervosa. It is dieting that usually appears to be the starting point for anorexia
nervosa.

Teens diet for a number of reasons. Sheila says she began
dieting to become a healthier person, whereas Tom's dieting was
initially designed to improve his diving. Most teenagers report
that dieting began because of a wish to lose weight, eat healthier,
or improve performance in a sport. A few adolescents begin consuming fewer calories in the service of being "good," as they
define it using an ascetic formulation along the lines of "The less
you consume, the better you are."

All of these motivations to diet share some common features. For example, each implies some notion of self-improvement,
in particular improvements that are concrete and outward and
thus noticeable by others—to look better, perform better, be
healthier. However, there are differences among these motivations for dieting as well. The emphasis on a thin appearance suggests a connection with social norms of beauty, whereas improvement in performance of a sport, in health, or in morality is
related more directly to perfectionism, drive, and ambition.
These latter qualities appear to be common personality features
in children who develop eating disorders.

Regardless of motivation, dieting usually begins informally. The child may start by cutting out desserts and snacks, but over time, meats and other proteins, fats, and sugars are eliminated too. Once food choices are narrowed, dieting efforts are typically focused on lowering the quantities of food consumed even within this limited range of options. Often detailed calorie counting, exact measuring, and elaborate preparation of foods become the rule. At this point adolescents may attempt to remove themselves from the company of others while eating, prepare meals independently of others, and sometimes cook elaborate meals and desserts for others without eating the food themselves.

Alongside this extreme food restriction, a schedule of increased exercise is often employed to ensure continued weight loss. At this point, whatever weight goals might have been set initially have typically been long surpassed, and the goal of weight loss in itself is firmly established. Sometimes self-induced vomiting or diet pill and laxative use may begin in an attempt to purge the small portions consumed.

For a child on the path to an eating disorder, eating is often associated with guilt, anxiety, and anger. Not eating, on the other hand, is associated with feelings of accomplishment, power, and strength. Paradoxically, with increased weight loss, hunger cues are diminished, making the process of continued food restriction easier. Nonetheless, most teens with anorexia are still extraordinarily preoccupied with food. Some will visit supermarkets and bakeries to look at and smell the food, but abstain from eating it. Parents may notice unusual food rituals beginning to develop, such as eating only out of certain bowls or plates, weighing and measuring foods precisely, using chopsticks, and so forth. The period of time over which this cascade of events takes place is variable, but it can be as short as 4–6 weeks or as long as a year or more. At some point during this process, in girls who have begun menses, menstruation likely ceases.

Sydney became too weak to swim and was taken off the swim team. At school, she was more and more isolated, and her friends stopped talking to her because they were afraid to ask her what was wrong. She became tearful and moody at home. She was so thin now that none of her clothes fit, even though they had been purchased only a month before, when school began. She was always cold; she wore sweaters and was constantly turning up the heat while the rest of the family sweltered. Her worried parents thought she was depressed and sought help from a psychiatrist.

FAILED DIETING AND OVEREATING: THE PATH TO BULIMIA NERVOSA

Sixteen-year-old Blair had always set high standards for herself. She wanted to be the best at everything. She worked hard at school and got good grades. She was generally well liked, though she always worried about who her friends were. She had worried about her weight for as long as she could remember and first began trying to lose weight when she went on a liquid diet with her mother when she was in fifth grade. She herself was never teased for being overweight, but she had seen other girls and boys teased when she was a child and was worried that she too would be teased. The diets she tried never made any difference. She lost a few pounds but then gained the weight back.

For the junior prom Blair decided she wanted to look great. She had a boyfriend, her first, and she wanted him to find her beautiful. That meant *thin*. Her boyfriend had never commented on her weight, but Blair was sure it was just because he was too nice to say anything. She knew she was too fat. She was determined to lose 15 pounds before the prom.

She began skipping breakfast altogether, and lunch as well. She would then go to the gym after school and exercise for 2 hours. She found some over-the-counter diet pills and drank lots of coffee, all in an effort to keep herself from being so hungry. Still, she woke up at night feeling hungry. But she stuck with her routine and lost 15 pounds for the prom. Everyone told her how wonderful she looked, and her boyfriend seemed happy with her appearance too. All of her friends congratulated her on her diet and wanted to know how she did it.

After the prom Blair tried to keep her diet plan going, but it became harder and harder to do. She would come home from school and be too tired to go to the gym. When she missed her workout, she was certain she would gain weight, so she tried to eat even less the next day. However, she began to be so hungry that she couldn't stop herself from eating. One day after school when no one else was home, Blair was so hungry that she ate a box of cookies. She went to the gym and tried to "exercise the calories she ate away," but there were too many and she was too tired. The same thing happened the next day. This time Blair was so upset she decided to try to throw up the cookies. She had promised herself that she would never do this, but she couldn't stand the worry about gaining weight. She would throw up just this once.

Blair tried to follow her own injunction, and sometimes she succeeded, but at least once or twice a week she failed and overate so much that she felt she had to purge. Slowly, week by week, she got into a pattern of eating very little and then binge eating in the afternoon, followed by purging. On days she found she couldn't vomit, she took some of her mother's laxatives to relieve her fears about gaining weight.

During this time, Blair's weight had gradually increased despite her efforts to diet, using diet pills and laxatives, and vomiting. Blair was increasingly despondent. Her boyfriend broke up with her because she stopped wanting to get together with him. She felt too ashamed of her weight to see him. In addition, she was afraid to go out with him because she might have to eat something and that would start her overeating.

Blair's mother hadn't suspected anything until one day she heard Blair throwing up in the shower. She asked her what was wrong, and Blair confessed to throwing up purposely, but only that one time. Still, her mother remained concerned and noticed that Blair had taken some laxatives from the medicine cabinet. Again, Blair denied she used them to lose weight, claiming she had done so because she was constipated. Finally, the mother of one of Blair's girlfriends called Blair's mother to tell her that her daughter had caught Blair throwing up at school. Blair's mother now tried to find help.

Binge-eating episodes and purging usually begin a little later than the extreme dieting of anorexia nervosa. Still, adolescents who binge eat and purge often report long histories of preoccupation with weight. Some say they remember worrying about their weight as early as kindergarten. Some were mildly to moderately obese during early childhood and remember being teased. Often these adolescents have experimented with a variety of diets for brief periods, only to abandon such efforts. Many report that in response to severe dieting and fasting behaviors, they develop an urge to overeat and feel increasingly out of control when eating. Once they've overeaten, they feel guilty and anxious and, as a result, seek ways to relieve themselves of their fear of gaining weight. This leads to purging in its various forms. Most often purging is accomplished through vomiting, but it can also include the use of laxatives, diuretics, and compensatory exercise.

Adolescents with bulimia nervosa, like their adult counterparts, report that to a great degree their self-worth depends on feeling satisfied with their weight and appearance. Often these adolescents report that they eat very little breakfast or lunch, but that upon returning to their homes after school, they binge. This is a time when there is usually little parental supervision and the binge eating can occur secretly. In addition, binge eating can become a way to cope with feelings of loneliness, boredom, and anxiety. Alternately, some adolescents report nighttime binge eating, another time when they are less likely to be observed.

Most adolescents, like adults, with bulimia nervosa report intense feelings of shame about these behaviors. As the disorder becomes more entrenched, teens begin to organize their lives around the management of binge eating and the compensatory activities related to it. They become more irritable and withdraw from friends and families. Often their schoolwork declines. They also report increasingly depressed moods. Once these altered patterns of eating are firmly established and extend their hold on the adolescent, binge eating and purging become a convenient way to avoid other problems and may be increasingly incorporated into the adolescent's coping strategies. These factors combine to make bulimia nervosa surprisingly resistant to change, even when someone is motivated to make such an effort. In addition, sometimes adolescents with bulimia nervosa report a history of other impulsive behaviors such as alcohol use and shoplifting.

Blair's mother took her to see a psychologist, who diagnosed her with bulimia nervosa, but Blair refused to return for therapy. Her mother tried to persuade her to go, but she said she could stop the behavior on her own. It appeared that this was the case, as Blair's mother saw no evidence of continued purging or binge eating for several months. However, her hopes were dashed when she discovered several bags of vomit and food containers in the garage. She called the psychologist again, who suggested they come in as a family to discuss how to proceed.

The first of the following lists contains items that you should be on the lookout for if you think it's possible your child is developing or has an eating disorder. If they are present, then you'll want to exercise additional vigilance to see if these warning signs are really indications that your child is developing an eating disorder that needs evaluation and treatment. The second list includes items that, if present, suggest that you need to take immediate action to have your child evaluated and treated.

WARNING SIGNS OF THE DEVELOPMENT OF AN EATING DISORDER

- Diet books
- Evidence of visiting pro-anorexia or eating disorder websites
- Dieting behavior
- Sudden decision to become a vegetarian
- Increased picky eating, especially eating only "healthy foods"

- Always going to the bathroom immediately after eating
- Multiple showers in a day (in order to purge in the shower), especially directly following eating
- Unusual number of stomach flu episodes
- Skipping meals
- Large amounts of food missing

ACT-NOW SIGNS AND SYMPTOMS

- Fasting and skipping meals regularly
- Refusing to eat with the family
- Two skipped periods (in girls) in conjunction with weight loss
- Any binge-eating episodes
- Any purging episodes
- Discovery of diet pills or laxatives
- Excessive exercise (more than an hour a day) and weight loss
- Persistent and unremitting refusal to eat nondiet foods
- Refusing to allow others to prepare foods
- Extreme calorie counting or portion control (weighing and measuring food amounts)
- Refusing to eat with friends

If at this point you've determined you need to have your child evaluated for an eating disorder, you'll want to consult someone who is an expert in these problems. This usually means someone besides a pediatrician or family physician, most of whom have had little training or experience with eating disorders. Certainly all of these professionals will have heard of eating disorders, and many will have had some limited experience, but most are not sure when an expert is needed, and they can unintentionally reassure parents, beyond the point at which they should, about not needing help.

This does not mean you should bypass your pediatrician or family physician on the way to an expert in eating disorders—quite the contrary. A physician can rule out other causes of your child's problems, which should get you closer to knowing whether an eating disorder is likely. Your pediatrician should be able to get an accurate weight and height for your child and perform a physical exam, including ordering basic laboratory work, that will uncover readily identifiable medical conditions that might be causing the problems you're observing—unexplained weight loss, loss of menstruation, or other physical symptoms such as lightheadedness or fainting. This examination may also reveal evidence that your child's problem is more urgent than you thought. If, for example, it turns out that your child has low blood pressure, a low heart rate, or signs of severe purging (erosion of tooth enamel, inexplicable swollen salivary glands, inexplicable weight loss), you'll know that you were right to act now. In some cases, when a teenager has developed such problems, hospitalization is necessary.

A basic medical workup for an adolescent with an eating disorder would include the following: a complete physical to check for signs of severe starvation (e.g., assessment of weight relative to height, low blood pressure, low heart rate, dry skin, low body temperature), as well as tests for liver, kidney, and thyroid functioning. These examinations help to assess the degree of illness and its chronicity, as well as to rule out other possible organic reasons for weight loss including diabetes, thyroid disease, or cancers. Common laboratory tests include a complete blood count; an electrocardiogram; studies of electrolytes, BUN (blood urea nitrogen), and creatinine; thyroid studies; and a test for urine specific gravity. Your pediatrician should be able to discuss the purpose of each of these tests, help you to understand any unusual laboratory results, and alert you if there is any cause for immediate medical intervention.

Assuming that your child is not too sick and that another medical problem is not clearly causing the problems with eating, you will need to proceed to an evaluation by an expert in eating disorders in children and adolescents. That's why you should take advantage of this appointment with the pediatrician to find out what kind of experience he or she has had with eating disorders. It may require a little tact and skill, but if you know the doctor fairly well, you will probably find a way to ask these important questions:

1. Have you seen many adolescents with eating disorders?
2. What do you recommend in terms of treatment (both medical and psychological)?
3. Whom do you refer your patients to and why?
4. How successful do you think your patients have been with treatment?

If your pediatrician proves not to be an expert, you can take steps to find one. We should note that pediatricians are sometimes reluctant to make referrals to such specialists because they are unsure whether changes in eating behaviors are due to emotional problems or just developmentally normal adolescent experimentation. In addition, because an adolescent with an eating disorder often denies or minimizes symptoms, physicians sometimes don't get the whole story from the adolescent. It might be helpful to go over the lists of warning signs presented earlier to encourage your pediatrician to make a referral if you have observed any of the behaviors on the "Act Now" list in your child.

A referral from your primary care physician or pediatrician often permits full insurance coverage for your child's psychiatric evaluation, so getting this referral rather than seeking an expert on your own is important for this reason as well. Scheduling such an evaluation may, unfortunately, be more complicated than it should be because of insurance processes and the limited availability of experts in eating disorders. Still, these obstacles can usually be overcome with persistence and a referral from a pediatrician specifying the need for the consultation.

Consult the Resources section at the end of this book for guidance on where to begin your search for help. One caveat, however: Many clinicians who treat adults with eating disorders are not prepared to evaluate younger patients. They are neither trained to look for the ways these younger patients' symptoms develop nor trained in ways to engage them or their parents in order to evaluate them effectively. There are many exceptions to this rule, of course, but the wise parent will inquire about the clinician's experience with younger patients before scheduling an appointment.

WHAT TO DO TO GET HELP

Most adolescents with eating disorders do not want help—at least initially. They see themselves as choosing to manage a problem with weight, and even if they recognize some problems with their dieting, they generally prefer to be left alone to sort it out themselves. Unfortunately, case descriptions like those you've just read make it pretty clear that many adolescents do not figure a way out soon enough to prevent serious problems from setting in. That leaves it up to parents to get the ball rolling sooner. This is easier said than done. So there are at least two problems parents face right away in trying to help their child with an eating disorder: (1) how to get their child to have an evaluation for an eating disorder and (2) whom and what to look for in terms of evaluation.

How to Get Your Child to Have an Evaluation

Before you delve into the challenge of getting your child to agree to an evaluation, make sure that you and your spouse (if there are two parents) agree that there is a problem that demands an evaluation. The importance of parents working together is a major theme of this book that is discussed in more detail later, particularly in Chapter 9. But even in agreeing that there is a problem, many parents differ on what to do about it. Using the guidelines provided in our lists of warning signs may help the two of you to see things the same way. And even if one parent is reluctant to move forward, the more concerned parent may have to take the lead initially to get things started. As long as the other parent doesn't manifest active opposition, this may be where some families have to start.

Once you're in agreement that your child needs a professional evaluation, it's important to let your child know you're planning to seek one. Springing the evaluation on her, which may be tempting inasmuch as you know she may resist going, can backfire because it makes it more likely that she will refuse to cooperate with the interviewer. Moreover, we feel it is important to be honest and up-front with your concerns. Deceiving your child about what you're doing makes it harder to develop trust, and ultimately you'll need that if you're going to be successful. Still, telling your child you're planning to seek professional help often leads to an uproar. Be prepared for your child to try to dissuade you from undertaking the consultation. Your child may object to missing school for the appointment or point out that you'll have to take time away from work, but you need to stand firm. The importance you place on this appointment sends a message that will be key to your continuing to be active in getting your child's problem under control. Certainly we have had parents "drag" their child in for an evaluation with us, but this is not the norm. Instead, a clear message that the pediatrician has made this referral, that you are concerned, and that this visit will help to clarify the situation is usually enough to get the child to the expert's clinic. Then it's up to the experts to do their job in providing a helpful assessment and set of treatment recommendations.

Whom and What to Look for in an Evaluation

Actually, in our experience, the second problem—getting a good evaluation for an eating disorder in a child or adolescent—is in some ways the greater problem of the two you face once you've decided you need help. Many communities don't have resources to assist with diagnosing and treating children and adolescents with eating disorders, particularly professionals who are up to date on the best techniques and approaches. It is clear that we cannot solve this problem with this book, but we hope that from the outset, by emphasizing the seriousness of the problems that eating disorders cause, we can encourage parents to make an effort to seek out regional expertise in the area, even if it is not available at the community level. We liken eating disorders to any other serious medical problem—such as leukemia or heart disease—for which it is often necessary to travel a bit farther to specialty centers for consultation and initial evaluation and treatment to achieve the best outcomes. In the Resources section of this book, we provide a guide to regional centers of expertise that we hope will help parents locate experts closer to them. At the same time, the following paragraphs provide a description of our evaluation process to help you know what to anticipate when you do have an expert consultation, based on processes at our treatment centers.

Once a referral has been made and an appropriate expert has agreed to meet with the patient and parents, an evaluation will probably begin with the clinician meeting alone with the adolescent. This provides a developmentally appropriate entry into the family that respects the adolescent's developing autonomy. The adolescent should expect to be interviewed with support and warmth, with the clinician minimizing presumptions of understanding. Open-ended questions about family, schoolwork, interests, and activities are used to break the ice with reluctant adolescents. Open-ended questions also provide an opportunity for the adolescent, when willing, to offer her own perspective on what's happening to her and what's motivating her and to express whatever level of discomfort she experiences with eating. This open-ended approach is also important because not presuming an understanding of what's happening, but still being clear about what needs to be explored, is the most objective way to gather information in a clinical interview.

It's important, of course, that the interview focus on eating behaviors and problems, but most clinicians will find that there is a significant amount of other relevant information to collect. This other information includes such things as medical problems, other behavioral issues (with adolescents this includes drug and alcohol use), perspectives on other family members, and any history of traumas or abuse. The interview identifies any history of concern about weight and shape or health that preceded the onset of dieting or other behavioral efforts to change weight and shape. Adolescents will be asked about their exposure to common triggers for dieting and weight concerns such as those mentioned earlier: hearing comments (positive or negative) on their weight, experiencing the onset of menses, dating, being involved in or exposed to family conflicts, starting middle school or high school, breaking up with a romantic partner, observing others beginning to diet at home or in their social circle, and so forth. The clinician should compile a detailed history about your child's efforts to lose weight. Examples of such behaviors include counting calories, restricting fat intake, fasting, skipping meals, restricting fluid intake, restricting meat and protein intake, increased or excessive exercising, binge eating, purging behaviors (exercise, use of laxatives or diuretics), and using stimulants and diet pills (over-the-counter items, health food products, and illegal products). Adolescents who binge eat and purge usually go through a cycle leading to increasing frequency of dieting, followed by binge eating and compensatory purgation. Persons with either anorexia or bulimia nervosa can binge eat and purge. However, those who are at extremely low weights who restrict their eating are more likely to call a much smaller quantity of food a "binge" than normal-weight adolescents who binge eat and purge.

Health consequences of these behaviors should also be evaluated. Adolescents with eating disorders commonly report chest pain, dizziness, headaches, fainting spells, weakness, poor concentration, stomach and abdominal pain, and loss of menses. For those with bulimia nervosa, throat pain, involuntary regurgitation, broken blood vessels in the eye, and swollen neck glands are also common. Because eating disorders are often accompanied by anxiety disorders, depression, personality disorders, or obsessive–compulsive disorder, the interviewer will ask about symptoms of these disorders as well.

In addition to those areas specific to eating problems, interviews will include an evaluation of other possible contributors to the development of the disorder, including physical and sexual abuse, traumas, and emotional and physical loss. Some elements of this aspect of the interview will be necessarily private and the contents not shared with you as parents unless warranted.

After the interview with the adolescent, you will usually be interviewed without your child present. If there are two of you, both of you need to be present. Your respective perspectives on your child and family are otherwise unavailable. You will be asked about the general development of your child—complications during pregnancy, early feeding, developmental milestones, transitions to preschool and elementary school, aspects of attachment (such as problems with separation when you dropped your child off at preschool, excessive clinging or irritable behavior when you were separated from your child, refusal to spend the night with friends because of fear of separation from you), early temperament and personality traits, family problems during childhood, and peer and sibling relationships. Your perspective on who your child is and how he or she may have come to have this problem creates an atmosphere of shared understanding and often makes it easier for the clinician to proceed to the specific history of the eating and weight problems that have brought you to the practitioner's office.

Next you will be asked how you saw the problem developing: When did you first perceive a problem? What have you tried to do to help? Do you see other kinds of emotional or developmental problems, such as depression or anxiety, peer problems, or other changes in behavior in your child? It's likely that the evaluation will compare information obtained during the interview with the adolescent with the parents' version of events and explore commonalities as well as differences. Together, these differing perspectives help generate a more comprehensive narrative of the events leading up to and sustaining the current eating problems.

Susan agreed to meet with the psychiatrist reluctantly. She did not want to miss school, and she said she was eating well. In the interview, Susan said she had lost weight because her stomach was bothering her—she had had the flu a few weeks ago, and her stomach was still recovering. She denied having any desire to lose weight and said she had eaten a muffin and juice for breakfast; a sandwich, chips, and cookies for lunch; and pasta with chicken and cheese sauce for dinner the day before. She said she exercised for only half an hour a day. She denied any lightheadedness, weakness, or headaches. She did admit to having skipped her menstrual period for the last 2 months.

When the clinician met with Susan's parents, they reported a very different version of events. Susan had begun losing weight about 5 months earlier. She did have the flu, but she had already lost 20 pounds by then and had lost another 5 pounds during that illness, which she had failed to gain back. Her parents reported that Susan had eaten about two bites of a muffin the morning before and drunk about 4 ounces of juice. They also said they had regularly found Susan's lunches in the trash. Susan also exercised for at least an hour a day and hardly ever sat down anymore.

Sometimes clinicians who treat eating disorders ask for consultation from a dietitian with expertise in working with eating disorders. Sometime dietitians calculate ideal body weight (IBW), which is derived from norms of weight for height in the patient's age group. Alternately, they may calculate the body mass index (BMI), defined as (weight in kilograms ÷ height in meters)². Either way, these weights serve as a general guide to determine a reasonable weight range for recovery. This can be helpful in clarifying the degree of weight loss your child has experienced and how far off he or she is from expected growth and weight norms for the child's age, maturity, and height. Dieticians can also provide educational advice to you, your teenager, and your doctors about the need for proper nutrition for health.

THE CHALLENGES OF DIAGNOSING AN EATING DISORDER

At the end of a proper consultation, if warranted, your child will likely receive a diagnosis of one of the major types of eating disorders. However, it is possible that the assessment will lead to a diagnosis of another problem that initially resembled, but is not, an eating disorder. Sometimes a fear of choking can lead to refusal to eat, and this may also look like anorexia. In this case, appropriate treatments would be for other conditions—depression and anxiety—rather than for an eating disorder.

Diagnoses are made to help clinicians decide on the best treatment recommendations for specific problems. So that you understand what the evaluating clinician means when rendering a diagnosis of your child, we think it is important that you know how eating disorders are described in the American Psychiatric Association's *Diagnostic and Statistical Manual of Mental Disorders*, the standard reference for diagnosing psychiatric problems in the United States.

Eating Disorder Diagnoses Overlap

Eating disorders are of three main types: *anorexia nervosa,*
bulimia nervosa, and *eating disorder not otherwise specified.* There
are differences among these three, but they also have many common features. We will be considering both these similarities and
differences in more detail later. The important thing to know
first is that it is sometimes difficult for a clinician to know at the
outset which of the three eating disorder diagnoses will be the
most accurate, because over time as many as one-third to one-
half of patients can be diagnosed with two or more of the different types of eating disorders. So, a good clinician will explain the
overlapping as well as distinguishing characteristics of the disorder types.

The Diagnostic Criteria Are Based on the Characteristics
of Adults with Eating Disorders

When we work with families, we like to stress that patients, and
adolescents in particular, do not necessarily conform to the criteria in a diagnostic manual. The *Diagnostic and Statistical Manual*
of Mental Disorders (also referred to as the DSM) has gone
through four full iterations in 30 years and is likely to continue
to evolve. That's because the DSM is based on increased clinical
knowledge about how mental diseases actually look. The DSM,
in general, takes adults as the model for how a mental illness
presents (exceptions include attention-deficit/hyperactivity disorder, pervasive developmental disorders, and oppositional defiant disorder, which are diseases that usually onset during childhood). In the case of eating disorders, the model used is clearly
an adult one. Although we discuss these diagnostic categories in
detail in Chapter 4, we want to emphasize here some of the
problems you will face with a younger child with an eating disorder because of the lack of developmental sensitivity in the DSM.

First, the weight criteria of 85% IBW or 17.5 BMI are problematic for older children and adolescents because they are
often still growing. Calculations used to derive these norms are
difficult to apply accurately in children who happen to be unusu-
ally tall, in boys, and in girls who have not yet reached the onset

of menses, leading to both under- and overestimations. The point is that using percentile weights may not be the best way to identify the child who has a serious eating problem of the anorexic type. Many patients who began serious dieting when they were significantly overweight are just as preoccupied and obsessed with continuing an unhealthy weight loss as those who more easily achieve these lower percentiles. In those cases, it is usually just a matter of time until they achieve these lower weights, but it is also precious time that has been lost when treatment should have begun.

Tony had been overweight his entire life. Both his mother and older sister were overweight as well. When Tony started eighth grade, he decided he would go on a diet. His parents supported this idea, because they felt it would improve his health and self-esteem. Tony was determined in his dieting and lost 10 pounds in a little more than 2 weeks by eating and drinking very little and beginning an exercise program of walking and jogging. Over the next 2 weeks, Tony increased his exercise and continued to eat very little. He lost another 5 pounds. He became increasingly focused on his dieting. He got up early in the morning to go for a run and stayed up late doing "crunches" and leg lifts. Over the next month, Tony lost another 5 pounds. He was now at a normal weight for his height, but his parents noticed that he was not satisfied. Tony said he wanted to lose another 20 pounds. Teachers reported that Tony was having trouble paying attention in class. Tony said he was just going over the calories he had eaten during that day. He was still getting good grades, but he no longer had time for friends because of his exercise program. His parents tried to get Tony to eat more, but he refused.

When Tony went to see a psychologist, he was told he had an eating disorder. Tony protested that he wasn't too thin and he wasn't throwing up his food. The psychologist pointed out that Tony was totally preoccupied with losing weight, food, counting calories, and excessive exercise. Tony countered that he was just "getting healthy" and that he was tired of being fat. Tony began to cry when told he needed help.

In addition to problems with weight loss criteria, menstrual criteria (i.e., three consecutive missed cycles) are difficult to apply in younger adolescents who have menstruated but who often have not firmly established periodic cycles. Moreover, there is no equivalent for males.

Fear of weight gain is also one of the cardinal features of anorexia nervosa in the DSM. However, for younger patients, it's often less clear to them what is motivating their restrictive eating, and many report not so much a desire to lose weight as the wish to be healthier, to be better performers in sport or dance, or to be better people by consuming less. In these cases, as in the case of Susan described earlier in this chapter, their behaviors speak more clearly than their stated intentions. In addition, younger patients tend not to report problems with how they perceive their bodies but instead deny, through their actions and sometimes words, the seriousness of their current low weight.

The criteria for bulimia nervosa do not allow even the few developmental concessions to adjust for age differences that are made for anorexia nervosa. Perhaps the most important problem with these criteria for adolescents with binge-eating and purging behaviors are the requirement of intensity (e.g., an average of twice a week) and the duration of symptoms (e.g., for 3 months). These reasonably apply to older, more chronic patients but pose significant problems for adolescents with binge-eating and purging behaviors earlier in the course of their illness. Symptoms of these types in adolescents may be intermittent, with varying intensities for briefer periods, and then quiescent. In addition, a slightly exaggerated focus on weight and shape may be somewhat normal for many adolescents, as may dieting and experimentation with various weight-loss strategies as a result. For parents, the trouble is that these criteria suggest that when a child doesn't meet these exact definitions the problem may not be serious. This is just not the case, as Tony's parents learned.

Because of the failure of the current DSM to capture early development of serious eating disorders, many children and adolescents are often best classified in the third category—eating disorder not otherwise specified, or EDNOS—if strict definitions of anorexia and bulimia nervosa are used. This can be helpful or confusing, depending on your perspective. To parents, EDNOS may seem vague and therefore dissatisfying; when you're worried about your child, you want the most definitive answers possible. To clinicians, the diagnosis may seem imprecise and therefore not as useful a guide to the correct treatment. If, however, you take a broader view of eating disorders and see what is common to anorexia and bulimia nervosa and EDNOS, rather than focus on how they are different, a diagnosis of EDNOS may be the most comprehensive and therefore allow clinicians to treat common elements of all eating disorders, such as excessive emphasis on the importance of weight and shape for self-worth and self-esteem and the pursuit of thinness through excessive dieting and other destructive weight loss procedures. From such a perspective, all persons with eating disorders share the following characteristics: a severely abnormal pattern of eating, an abnormal attitude or set of beliefs about food, weight, and/or shape, a degree of emotional, social, or behavioral dysfunction resulting from these behaviors and attitudes (significant problems with school, work, social or familial functioning), and evidence that these behaviors and attitudes are very unlikely to change without intervention. This was certainly the case for Tony, who received a diagnosis of EDNOS initially but might have gone on to develop anorexia or bulimia nervosa over time if his parents hadn't gotten help early on. EDNOS can be every bit as serious as anorexia nervosa or bulimia nervosa. Just because someone doesn't fit in the boxes doesn't mean the problem isn't as bad. Unfortunately, some parents and clinicians miss this fact and delay treatment even though the evidence is compelling that big problems with eating already exist.

In summary, the current traditional diagnostic categories of anorexia and bulimia nervosa apply to only some of the children and adolescents seen with eating problems severe enough to warrant professional help. Nonetheless, the current diagnostic system is what you will face when you try to understand if and what kind of eating disorder your child may have. So it is important that you keep these limitations in mind, because they suggest that a diagnosis alone may be insufficient to guide you in understanding what to do next. However, as we show throughout this book, there is growing evidence that your active participation is key to resolving many of the problems that these disorders have in common.

Although you will be faced with the dilemma of how to get started, as we've described here, you should be less uncertain about when to act. Now is the time. The one thing you can be certain of is that once eating disorders become established, they do not give up their firm emotional and physical grip on your child. We know that for both anorexia and bulimia nervosa the longer someone has the illness, the more difficult it is to treat. For anorexia, for example, we have little evidence, of any effective treatments after someone has been ill for more than a few years. In the case of bulimia we know that a chronic course, in which symptoms come and go for periods of several years, is a common pattern when the illness goes untreated. A delay in taking action only facilitates increased habituation to these illnesses, making it harder for you to succeed in helping your child. So act now!

FOR MORE INFORMATION

American Psychiatric Association, *Diagnostic and Statistical Manual of Mental Disorders*, Fourth Edition, Text Revision, 2000. Washington, DC: American Psychiatric Association.

Fairburn, C. G., and K. D. Brownell, Editors, *Eating Disorders and Obesity: A Comprehensive Handbook*, Second Edition, 2002. New York: Guilford Press.

Garner, D. M., and P. E. Garfinkel, Editors, *Handbook of Treatment for Eating Disorders*, Second Edition, 1997. New York: Guilford Press.

Natenshon, A. H., *When Your Child Has an Eating Disorder: A Step-by-Step Workbook for Parents and Other Caregivers*, 1999. San Francisco: Jossey-Bass.

Thompson, J. K., *Handbook of Eating Disorders and Obesity*, 2004. Hoboken, NJ: Wiley.

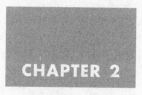

CHAPTER 2

GET TOGETHER

Everyone is confused.

Bridget refused to eat with her family. Her mother told her father that Bridget was going through a phase. She just needed time to make her own decisions. Bridget's father disagreed. He felt she was stonewalling the family and shouldn't be treated differently from anyone else. Bridget's sister was mad that she still had to eat dinner with her parents and little brother. Bridget's little brother said he missed Bridget and asked how come she didn't eat with them now.

No one knows what to do.

Myra has had anorexia nervosa for 2 years now. She meets with her therapist twice a week and her nutritionist once a week. Myra says her therapist tells her that she needs to decide to eat and get better and that her parents should stay out of it. The therapist said as much to her parents as well. The nutritionist advises Myra on what to eat and how much. Myra's parents aren't sure what Myra's weight is or what the nutritionist is recommending, but Myra remains very thin and her food choices quite limited.

You are frightened and angry.

> For the third time this week, Sam is making a trip to the bathroom just after eating dinner. Sam's father follows him to the bathroom at a safe distance. Through the closed door Sam's father hears the shower being turned on, and a few minutes later he hears a coughing and choking sound. Sam's father stands outside the door and begins to cry silently.

You've been told by therapists and friends and you've read in books and on Internet websites that if your child has an eating disorder, you should stay out of it and let the therapist help your child work on the issue. You're told that this hands-off approach is the correct one, because a salient feature of eating disorders is the need to control something. Adolescents with eating disorders reportedly feel "out of control," and it follows that this makes them feel anxious, so they seek to control the one thing they think they can control—what they eat. You've also been told that these feelings of being out of control probably arise from things you did as a parent. You were either too intrusive and overinvolved and controlling, or too distant, underinvolved, and abusive. Either way, you're the source of the problem, and therefore you can't be part of the solution. In fact, the farther away you are, the better.

You've heard all these things, but they don't feel right to you. How can you stand by and watch your daughter starve herself or listen outside the bathroom door while your son throws up his dinner? How do you explain to your other children that you know their brother or sister is not eating or is binge eating or is throwing up, but that you're trying to help by letting their sibling "manage" it alone? They don't buy it. Your other children are already trying to get your son to eat more and to quit throwing up. These things don't feel right to you because your gut sense as a parent is that it is somehow wrong to stand by and do nothing when one of your children is suffering. It also doesn't make sense to you because you know that you should be able to help. You *need* to help.

Why is it so hard to find a way to help with eating disorders? You would know what to do if your child had another kind of problem, even a very serious one like cancer—you'd take him or her to the hospital, get the best doctors, support your son or daughter during radiation therapy, surgery, or chemotherapy by being with the child. You would make sure that you understood the medicines, and you would make sure your child took them. You would make sure your daughter or son got to all scheduled appointments for follow-up visits, and you'd be on the lookout for signs of relapse or problems.

In other words, you would be a part of helping, no matter what. You would take off work or quit work if needed. You would borrow money to pay for treatment. You would question the doctors, and you would carefully evaluate all of their recommendations. You would not leave all decisions up to your child, because you know that your child wouldn't or couldn't fully appreciate the repercussions of complicated decisions and options. You would do these things because you are a parent.

In contrast, when your child has an eating disorder, you are often left to your own devices. You don't know what's being done in terms of treatment. You're not sure about what options there are. You are told not to interfere with the therapist's and nutritionist's recommendations. You are told to butt out.

After her third hospitalization in 5 months for a low heart rate and blood pressure due to starvation, 13-year-old Sarah's parents were fed up. Each time Sarah came home she had promised to eat more. There were always excuses. Sarah's therapist felt she wasn't trying in therapy. Sarah's nutritionist said she wouldn't see her anymore unless she agreed to eat more and gained weight. Sarah's pediatrician felt she should be sent to a residential treatment center, where she would get 24-hour-a-day care, individual therapy, group therapy, dance therapy, pet therapy, recreational therapy, medications, and art therapy. Her parents would be 500 miles away. Sarah didn't want to be sent away. She was trying her best.

You wonder why eating disorders are so different from other illnesses. Why shouldn't you be able to help? Isn't there a way to help? There *must* be a way to help.

There *is* a way to help.

HOW THE NATURE OF EATING DISORDERS PITS PARENTS AGAINST THEIR CHILDREN

You know that your son or daughter has changed since developing an eating disorder. You've observed that your child is more distant, seems depressed or moody or irritable, is obsessive about food (and probably other things). In some cases the teen's already pronounced tendencies toward perfectionism are further accentuated. Actually, your child's driven nature is more pronounced, period, whether in a good way or a bad way. What has happened?

We like to use a Venn diagram to describe what has happened (see Figure 1). One circle (white) represents your child before the eating disorder started. The other (black) represents the eating disorder. Over time, the eating disorder circle increasingly overlays the circle that represents your child. Her circle pattern is still there and recognizable but is now being altered by the eating disorder. So, many of her traits, although still present, are colored by the eating disorder. Say, for example, she tends to be perfectionistic. This trait is still present, but now it is particularly evident in connection with food—precise calorie counting, exact measuring, obsessive label reading, and so forth. Or perhaps she is anxious. Now her anxiety is increased at mealtime, and she refuses to eat around family or friends. Driven qualities can also be redirected. She now exercises for 3 or 4 hours a day at increasingly intense levels. We like to say that the eating disorder is using your child's characteristics (often great strengths)

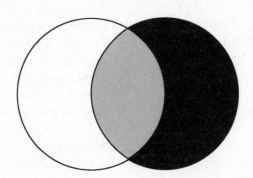

FIGURE 1. How an eating disorder overshadows your child's true self.

against her. That's one of the reasons it's so hard for your child to battle the illness on her own—she's fighting herself and her own determination, drive, perfectionism, and obsessiveness. This combination of your child's characteristics and those of the eating disorder is confusing. You recognize your child's personality traits, and yet there are these major changes in focus—about food, weight, and exercise. This makes it difficult to know how to proceed. Some of the very things you may value in your child now stand in the way of your being able to help her. Here's an example: Your child is an exceptionally talented ballet dancer. She develops anorexia nervosa. You see her losing weight, but she gets a principal role in the dance company's production. Her talent, persistence, and ambition are paying off, but they are also being used to further the physical and emotional devastation of anorexia nervosa. As a parent you're torn between supporting your child's talent and allowing anorexia nervosa to become further entrenched.

Maybe that example is too easy. Suppose your daughter is a high school marathon runner. She is likely to be one of the best in the state. However, she has started throwing up and not eating so as to improve her performance. Her performance does improve. Still, she exercises more and more. Her performance begins to deteriorate. You know she has an eating disorder and should quit the team, but your daughter cries that without running she will get depressed and will kill herself. That's all she cares about.

Here's yet another example: Your child is preparing for the SAT. She's gotten straight A's and is taking AP (advanced placement) courses. Her SAT scores, though, are not as high as they need to be to clinch her admission to the prestigious college she aspires to. In addition to having anorexia, she has become an overdedicated student—staying up very late at night and getting up very early—in preparation for retaking the SAT, which is about 8 months away. You see that her focus on schoolwork is actually helping to prevent her from eating normally, and you hear her exercising late at night when she's taking a break. She tells you she has to study for the SAT and needs to exercise to keep awake. You want her to get into the college she wishes to attend, but you also see her becoming thinner, with darker circles under her eyes, and increasingly withdrawn from friends and family.

All of the preceding examples demonstrate how the nature of eating disorders is confusing for parents and can pit them against their child. However, there are other ways that eating disorder symptoms lead to conflicts between parents and children. One of the most bedeviling problems is the timing of these illnesses. They usually occur just when adolescents are both more able to be independent and certainly very interested in being so. Thus, you are battling both the symptoms of the illness and the developmentally appropriate stage of increasing independence. In other words, sometimes you don't know if you're struggling with an eating disorder or with typical adolescent strivings for autonomy. When your child says to you, "I'm old enough to make my own decisions about what I eat," there is a ring of truth to it. The only problem is that often when adolescents make decisions because they have an eating disorder, and battle for them, the fight is "fixed"—the eating disorder wins and both you and your child lose.

> Lidia had always been fiercely independent. When she was a preschooler, she spent hours learning to tie her shoes rather than let someone help her. Her parents had always respected Lidia's spirit and supported her when she struggled with the task, because they could understand what she was trying to accomplish on her own. As a young teenager, Lidia had chosen her own classes, decided who her friends would be, and chosen her own clothes. Not surprisingly, when she began losing weight and her parents tried to step in to help her, Lidia was strident in her opposition. She fought over every morsel, filled herself up with water, and refused to eat anything her mother cooked for fear that her mother had put butter in it. At first her parents chalked this up to normal teenage rebellion and delayed taking any definite action about treatment. Lidia continued to lose weight and then began binge eating and purging. Now they realized that the things they were fighting Lidia about were not normal teenage issues, nor were they rational problems. They were evidence that Lidia's thinking had gone awry and that an eating disorder had developed.

Along with this striving for independence, with adolescence come increased wishes for privacy. This too helps eating disorders along. Eating disorders tend to increase secretive behaviors to avoid detection and thereby prevent intervention. So, because of others' respect for these adolescent needs for privacy, eating disorders can go on for months and even years without anyone really appreciating their presence. This is true despite the fact that adolescents themselves often leave abundant clues. Some save all the packages from the food they consume in boxes under their beds. Others vomit into plastic containers and save them in their closets. Still others lose a great deal of weight and hide under sweatshirts and baggy clothes. Even if you've noticed some of these behaviors, it feels like prying to ask about them. Such is the power of an adolescent's need for privacy.

It's pretty clear that the symptoms of eating disorders, your child's personality traits, and the expectations for autonomy and privacy during adolescence make it difficult to know how to take this problem on. How can you?

HOW CURRENT APPROACHES TO TREATMENT CAN REINFORCE CONFUSION ABOUT THE FAMILY'S ROLE

The main approaches to treating adolescents with eating disorders are family therapy and individual psychodynamic therapy (discussed in more detail later in this book). These two approaches are important clinical interventions that undoubtedly help many adolescents with eating disorders. At the same time, some of the ways these two approaches conceive of parental involvement can be problematic both for your child and for you as a parent.

There are long-standing debates about the role of parents in the treatment of anorexia nervosa. The earliest physicians to describe the treatment of anorexia nervosa disagreed about this. In the late 19th century, Charles Lasegue in France felt parents were essential to treatment, whereas Sir William Gull, just across the English Channel, proposed that parents were the "worst attendants." Many current approaches either exclude or blame parents, explicitly or implicitly, causing parents to be confused about whether and how they can help their child with an eating disorder. In addition, because of the severity of both the psychiatric and medical problems of anorexia nervosa, hospitalization or residential care is often recommended. This requires separating the child with anorexia nervosa from you and other family members. "Parentectomy" is seen as desirable and is still common in Europe, though the costs of these types of long-term hospitalization have become very burdensome in the United States.

Short of a parentectomy, some individual approaches to the treatment of adolescents with eating disorders in the outpatient setting also advise strongly against parental involvement. These approaches view the young adolescent with anorexia nervosa as having an inadequate sense of self resulting from a problematic relationship with her parents, usually her mother. This inadequate sense of self is supposedly due to insufficient nurture and respect for the child's needs and failure to sufficiently separate maternal needs from those of the developing child. These developmental failures lead to the child's developing an identity based on overcompliance with parents' and other authorities' expectations, with little sense of her own needs and wishes. During adolescence this compliant strategy falters, but because of fear of parental rejection, feelings of powerlessness, and little sense of her real wishes, the teenager turns to extreme dieting and an irrational pursuit of thinness as a way of expressing her internal anxieties about separation and individuation. She feels "out of control" because she does not have the internal resources to cope with the independent thought and action required during adolescence and adulthood. A focus on what she can control, her weight and food intake, provides reassurance that she has some identity—albeit one devoted to the sole pursuit of thinness. In this way anorexia nervosa becomes intricately bound up with the developing sense of identity, making it difficult to challenge.

Certainly many adolescents with anorexia nervosa do seem to struggle with the typical adolescent issues. Nonetheless, the implication that treatment should be focused only on the adolescent through her relationship with a therapist to "re-parent" her is questionable on several grounds. First, there is little scientific evidence supporting the notion that parents, and mothers in particular, of children with anorexia nervosa, systematically differ from others in how they have parented their children. Most parents of children who develop anorexia nervosa have other kids who do not develop the disorder but were generally parented similarly. Studies of the feeding practices of mothers whose children later develop anorexia nervosa show that they don't appear to differ substantially from typical feeding practices. For example, although one researcher found that "picky eating and early introduction of solid foods" predicted more eating disorders in adolescence, these same practices when used with siblings did not lead to eating difficulties. Further, studies of parental psychopathology as an indicator of overinvolvement with children don't provide clear evidence that these parents truly differ from others. The studies suggesting that this is the case evaluated families who were in crisis about their child's starving, making it impossible to draw conclusions about their functioning without this stress. In other words, even those studies that find evidence of intrusiveness and overinvolvement in families in which a child has an eating disorder can only say that these differences were present once an eating disorder had developed, but not before. This is important, because it is this presumption—that parents, in particular mothers, have *caused* the problem of anorexia nervosa in their children—that supports the clinical notion that they should be excluded from treatment.

Gabe was always good at school, though he was somewhat shy. He didn't really like rough sports, but he excelled at tennis and swimming. When he developed anorexia nervosa at age 14, his parents took him to a psychiatrist who said he believed that Gabe was struggling with being independent and was confused emotionally and sexually. The psychiatrist suggested psychoanalysis as a way to help Gabe address these problems instead of avoiding them by starving himself. His parents wanted only the best for their son, and they had the resources to pay for intensive psychotherapy—anything to help him.

Gabe was happy enough at first to go to therapy. He was never a disobedient child. Even as a teenager, he seldom mouthed off or complained about his parents' requests. However, over time Gabe complained about time away from his homework (he was in an honors class in all subjects) and from his workout schedule, which included a 2-hour swim in the morning and a run in the afternoon. He said he liked this therapist. They talked about his friends and his parents, but not much about eating or weight.

His parents dutifully took Gabe to therapy four afternoons a week However, after a few months, they didn't see any improvement. In fact, they felt Gabe was getting worse. He was still losing weight and eating even less. His therapist had told them to let Gabe decide what to eat and when to exercise, and they deferred to this recommendation, though they were constantly worried. Things came to a head when Gabe began to refuse to go to therapy. He said that he didn't see any reason to go and that he was better. His parents could see that he wasn't.

Other adherents of individual therapy have excluded parents for developmental reasons. Developmental theorists have suggested that to support adolescent autonomy, parents should be, in the main, left out of treatment. To support age-appropriate autonomy, some clinicians contend that it is the adolescent herself who must take on the challenge of anorexia nervosa, more or less as a preamble to beginning to emerge as an adolescent once again. Parents will, according to this school of thought, simply reinforce the preadolescent stance, furthering the regressive hold that anorexia nervosa has on their child.

Gary was on his high school's rowing crew and had developed anorexia nervosa initially while trying to be as fit and as lean as possible to better succeed at this sport. When Gary's parents took him to a therapist, she suggested that Gary was struggling with a wish to be more independent but was frightened of the responsibilities of work and relationships that being more grown up would entail. She suggested that Gary needed help with being more self-assertive and that he should be given more control over his life as was appropriate for a 16-year-old boy. Gary's parents agreed that he should be independent, but they thought at this point he was too ill to make good decisions and were worried about the consequences to his health if he made poorer ones. Risk

taking and exploration are a part of adolescence, the therapist explained, and it was necessary to trust Gary more and
let him make mistakes if need be.

Gary competed avidly on crew and his team did well, but
by midseason he was no longer able to participate because
he had lost additional muscle mass and wasn't strong enough
to row even short distances. Gary said he understood that he
had made a mistake and would now eat more to gain his
muscle back. He did this for a while but became anxious
about getting out of shape and once again cut back on eating and increased his exercise. Gary's parents wanted to step
in to help their son, but because they wished to respect his
adolescent need for independence, they held back.

You only have to think about the behavior of children with
anorexia nervosa to see that the illness effectively stops adolescent development. It throws children off the normal trajectory
of physical maturation (ceasing menstruation, for example),
encourages them to isolate themselves from the peers with
whom they need to start to align to acquire independence, and
leads to their being more involved with their parents and family,
because of being ill, than would be usual for a teenager. But why
would this necessarily lead to a conclusion that adolescents with
anorexia nervosa should face the challenge of battling this illness
without a great deal of parental involvement? After all, kids
don't generally face the challenges of adolescence without parents. In fact, the presumption that having a stormy, conflict-
ridden relationship with their parents is a necessary rite of passage for all teenagers, no longer has much support. We now
know that the teenagers who function best are those who continue to make productive use of their parents during adolescence—whose parents develop skills that enhance and support
their adolescent children's progress through this stage of bur-
geoning autonomy. This may be even truer for adolescents who
have difficulties of one kind or another. That is, teenagers who
not only face the predictable challenges of adolescence but also
have a physical or emotional problem are likely to need to rely
even more on parental resources to ensure their ultimate success
with and mastery of the tasks of adolescence. Thus, it may be all

the more important for teenagers who develop anorexia nervosa to be able to garner the support of their parents in their struggles with the illness.

Many of the core features of eating disorders are also seen by some as requiring the dilemmas they present to be faced by the individual patient in individual therapy rather than through parental management. Eating disorders are often described as illnesses of "control," and so it is assumed that "taking control" away from the adolescent in regard to eating and dieting will exacerbate the problem. It's true that eating disorders lead to high levels of anxiety about food and weight, and indeed this anxiety decreases, relatively but briefly, when patients feel they are controlling these parts of their lives. Nonetheless, the anxiety returns rapidly and with renewed insistence, leading to even greater restriction and control, resulting in a cascade of increasing weight loss and worry. Patients report their mind-numbing preoccupations with counting calories, reading recipes, counting fat grams, weighing, measuring, special cookware, plates, and so on. The misery that accompanies these preoccupations is tolerable only because of the relief from the anxiety, which occurs intermittently, that reinforces these behaviors.

However, if eating disorders are diseases of control, the sense of control is quite illusory. Patients do not feel in control; rather, they feel a need to feel in control. This difference is crucial. The pursuit of thinness, weight loss, dieting, and so forth, is a search for control, not true evidence of control. In this sense, contending that the adolescent needs to remain in control of her eating and diet is a fabrication, because when she has an eating disorder she does not have this control to begin with; instead, she is constantly trying to reassure herself that she will get such control. In this sense, the adolescent with an eating disorder is in need of someone to take control or at least help her take control, rather than leave her with an ever-shrinking ability to meet the behavioral and psychological demands of her illness.

Ironically, treatment modalities that advocate parentectomy to a greater or lesser extent, in the name of giving the adolescent control over food and weight, actually take most of the control away. Hospital programs regularly insist on consumption of set amounts of food or liquid supplements over which the patient exercises no control. Dietitians regularly prescribe dietary regimens for patients to follow. Some refeeding programs (professionally administered programs designed to rapidly restore weight) simply resort to nasogastric refeeding rather than involve the patient in even the activity of chewing and swallowing. Still, upon discharge, parents are told to let the child manage her food choices on her own. What is interesting, though, is that most younger patients experience a brief period of relief of anxiety when they are treated in such programs. That is, when someone else takes control of their eating and weight, they can often allow themselves to let go of the anxiety about these concerns. This accounts to no small degree for the success of these inpatient refeeding programs in treating the acute weight loss and malnutrition associated with anorexia nervosa. If most people with an eating disorder simply rejected these interventions, these programs would not succeed.

Why don't people with eating disorders rebel against these intrusive procedures as they do at home? It could be argued that it is against their nature to be confrontational and directly rebellious. Others report that these people have supreme (and somewhat justifiable) confidence that they can undo this weight gain rather quickly once they are allowed to be in charge again. Both of these perspectives are likely true, but certainly the latter point is not contested. Though most refeeding programs succeed in helping people with anorexia to eat more in the hospital (or other intensive settings), many lose the weight gained and revert to their restrictive behaviors when left to their own devices upon discharge. The question then is how best to build on the progress accomplished in these programs.

Lilly was a precocious 10-year-old who developed anorexia after she lost weight at summer camp. She was hospitalized for severe starvation. In the hospital, Lilly at first protested against eating and yelled and cried for her mother. She complained about missing her family and her friends. She hated missing school. Members of the nursing staff, who were quite experienced with these behaviors, provided a consistent presence at mealtimes and quietly insisted that Lilly eat her meals. They waited with her, encouraged her when needed, and set a limit on how long she had to complete her meals. Meals were provided at regular intervals, and snacks were also served routinely. Lilly gained weight and seemed less troubled by her eating symptoms, and after 3 weeks was discharged home.

Lilly almost immediately began to restrict her eating again. Her parents were unsure what to do, although they now knew more about anorexia nervosa than they had before. Lilly said that she and the nutritionist had worked out a meal plan that she was supposed to follow. Her parents didn't really understand it. Meanwhile, Lilly started school immediately and threw herself into the work with her usual vigor. As she studied more and once again became preoccupied with her grades, she ate even less. Within 2 months Lilly was back in the hospital, weighing even less than she had when she was first admitted.

Another reason parents have been excluded from individual treatment is the assumption that parents of adolescents with eating disorders are unduly focused on weight and dieting. The theory is, somewhat reasonably, that parents are the vehicle through which children and adolescents learn about and filter their experiences of the culturally informed thin ideal. Parents who emphasize extreme concerns about weight in themselves, others, or their children are seen as likely to promote body dissatisfaction in their children, who internalize the thin ideal as communicated by their parents. For this reason, treatments focused on helping with body image dissatisfaction or, more important, body image distortion, exclude parents, who are seen as the likely suspects in causing this increased reliance on the thin ideal as a source of self-evaluation. Although it is undoubtedly true that parents can influence dieting concerns and behaviors, few support the distortions associated with eating disorders even if they have the illness themselves. Instead, parents can and often do serve as a reality check on these distortions and thereby likely mediate the influence of other social and cultural pressures such as the use of alcohol and drugs, sexual activity, and social role performance.

Yet another reason that you may be excluded from treatment is that many therapists believe that you have caused the illness or are doing things to make it worse. Families themselves have been implicated in the etiology and maintenance of
anorexia nervosa. The most famous formulation of the family as
the cause of anorexia nervosa is based on the psychosomatic
family process as observed by Salvador Minuchin and colleagues.
These clinical investigators characterized psychosomatic families
(including families with a child with anorexia nervosa) as enmeshed, overprotective, conflict avoidant, and rigid and said
that each characteristic led to difficulties for the adolescent in
negotiating the transition to adolescence:

1. In enmeshed families, the needs of the individual were
   unclear and difficult to assert.
2. Overprotective families prevented adolescents from the
   necessary social and psychological risk taking crucial for
   developing autonomy.
3. Families that tended to avoid conflict thwarted the necessary strivings for independent thinking and behavior.
4. Rigid families had difficulty adapting to the necessary
   change in role and function associated with having an
   adolescent whose needs were different from those of
   younger children.

In addition to these problems in family process, psychosomatic
families were said to have structural problems, such as where
children take up the role of a parental figure and/or where the
parents, facing the developmental challenges of adolescence,
abdicate responsibility. Other researchers have suggested that
there may be problems in how parents are emotionally connect-
ed (attached) to their children with anorexia nervosa. Some feel
these parents promote a kind of false independence by not relat-
ing sincerely and deeply to their children. If children develop
this "false independence," it tends not to hold up during adolescence, and problems such as eating disorders may ensue.

Monica and her family came to family therapy for anorexia nervosa after they had read that problems in families

were often the reason children developed eating disorders. Monica's parents were professionals who had accomplished a lot in their respective careers. Her father was an accountant who traveled a great deal, and her mother was a real estate agent. There were no other children. Monica had been a somewhat anxious child, but over time she had gained increasing confidence and had, to all appearances, sailed through elementary school both academically and socially. When she developed anorexia nervosa in eighth grade, it was the parents' first sign that there were problems.

The family met with the therapist, who determined that Monica was too close to her parents, particularly her mother. Being too close to her mother interfered with Monica's need to be more independent as a teenager. In addition, and in part because Monica and her mother were so close, Monica's father and mother, it was suggested, weren't acting together, and instead Monica was usurping her father's role. Finally, the therapist said, the family needed to address their suppressed anger. They needed to acknowledge their disagreements with one another. The family agreed to try.

For several weeks the therapist asked the family to describe their conflicts, which were at this point all about Monica's not eating. The therapist accepted that not eating was the subject of their arguments but suggested that not eating was just a symptom of other conflicts they weren't describing. The family was increasingly perplexed but tried hard to identify problems. Monica's parents spent more time together, as the therapist directed. Monica was encouraged to spend time outside the family, which she did, mostly by going on runs or going to the gym. Meanwhile, Monica continued to lose weight and had gone on to her eighth month without a menstrual period. Monica's parents asked the therapist when they could expect Monica to get better.

The research literature on the pathology of parents and families of adolescents with anorexia nervosa is fraught with difficulties, and conclusions are far from clear. Many researchers and clinicians argue that it is not the family that is causing some of the problematic behaviors seen in teens with anorexia nervosa, but rather the illness and the family's experiences of the illness. In other words, families become overprotective *because* their children are ill. They become enmeshed *because* they're trying to understand what's happening to their child and therefore appear intrusive and overinvolved. They want to avoid conflicts *because* they fear making things worse. They become more rigid *in reaction* to the stress the illness imposes on them. Although this debate is not resolved, the position taken by many clinicians is to presume the parents and family are guilty until proven innocent, thereby justifying the limitation of parental involvement in treatment.

Despite this stance by many clinicians, the notion that parents are unnecessary to treatment has been challenged increasingly over the years. Family therapists view the families of patients with anorexia nervosa as not only necessary to involve in treatment but essential to the recovery process. However, many still arrive at that conclusion because they see families as the "problem" in anorexia nervosa, and therefore neglecting to treat them would mean leaving the essential core of the illness to fester. It is only recently that parents and families of adolescents with anorexia nervosa have been perceived as being likely to exert a *positive influence* on bringing about recovery of anorexia nervosa but *not* being perceived as the likely cause of the problem to begin with.

HOW FAMILIES CAN COME TOGETHER TO FIGHT EATING DISORDERS

As we've said, many current therapies exclude parents and families, pay them only lip service, or blame them for causing or worsening the illness. However, there is another therapeutic approach that takes a different view. First developed at the Maudsley Hospital in London, this form of family therapy doesn't blame the family but encourages its members to support their child actively by taking responsibility for refeeding the child. This treatment, unlike many of the other currently used approaches, has been actually studied in a series of trials that provide evidence that it is helpful. Indeed, it's the only therapy for anorexia nervosa that has any substantive empirical support (see Chapter 6).

The basics of what's called the Maudsley approach are as follows. First, parents and the family as a whole are helped to understand how serious eating disorders are. To do this, the therapist reviews just how much the adolescent has changed, as well as the trajectory of serious problems (medical and psychological) that follow if the eating disorder goes unchecked. Next, the therapist helps family members to see how important they are in changing the outcome, while reminding them of their abilities and previous successes in solving other family problems. The therapist also reminds parents that unless they are prepared to send their child away, it will be they who ultimately have to be responsible for setting up an environment that supports improved behaviors related to eating and weight. This can feel overwhelming, and so parents are assured that the therapist will help them, not by telling them what to do, but rather by reviewing with them their successes and dilemmas and problem solving with them, using the resources that parents and siblings bring to help.

With this as an impetus, the therapist, using his or her expertise and experience, consults with parents in their efforts to change maladaptive eating behaviors. When working together with a therapist, most parents are able to make dramatic changes in such behaviors relatively quickly. When these behaviors have ceased to be the main concern, the therapist encourages the parents to help their adolescent manage eating independently, but with some guidance. Once the adolescent is managing eating and weight on her own, the therapist concludes treatment by strategizing with the family members about how they might address more general issues of adolescence. This helps to prepare the family to leave therapy ready to proceed in the normal course of things.

We've been using this therapy in our centers for eating disorders in adolescents for a number of years now. We have been involved in research, as well as in clinical work using this approach that doesn't blame parents, but helps them better help their children with the symptoms of eating disorders and provides ample opportunity for education and support. Consequently, we've seen adolescents with eating disorders improve dramatically. Not only do their symptoms abate, but, on the whole, the family also feels better able to negotiate adolescent issues in other areas.

Even if this form of family therapy is not available to your child, adopting its principles, described in the following paragraphs, can help you find a way to be involved in your child's treatment, to the child's ultimate benefit.

1. **Parents bring important resources to their child's recovery and can be involved in whatever type of treatment the child receives.** It's the purpose of this book, in fact, to demonstrate how you can adopt this perspective to your child's benefit in a variety of clinical settings.

2. **It's important for parents to take eating disorders seriously.** One of the insights that the Maudsley approach highlights is the importance of realizing that eating disorders are serious medical and psychiatric illnesses. They are so serious, in fact, that as a parent you need to be highly aware of their potential for killing or severely damaging your child. Bulimia nervosa and anorexia nervosa are not just instances of taking dieting too far; they are truly *illnesses*. By emphasizing this principle, as we began to do in Chapter 1, we hope to help motivate you to take more immediate and definite action to help your child.

3. **You need to know what you're up against.** As a parent, you need to become sufficiently informed about the eating disorders that you know how to evaluate to a reasonable degree whether your child is getting better or not doing well. Parents are prepared for many difficulties that adolescents may develop, but they are understandably not expected to know very much about eating disorders. The work by the Maudsley group, as well as that in our own centers, demonstrates that educating parents about how people with eating disorders think and behave, and why they do the odd things they do, helps parents to be more sympathetic, supportive, and effective in helping their children.

4. **It's not your fault.** Our approach includes a nonblaming attitude toward parents. If you feel guilty and responsible for causing the eating disorder, you likely also feel hopeless and inadequate when facing the task of trying to help your child change her eating behaviors. As we've said, though, we believe

you are a key ingredient to your child's success in fighting the eating disorder. So it's our job, both in our practice and in this book, to alleviate any anxiety or guilt that is keeping you from contributing to your child's return to health.

5. **You need to be empowered to take up your parental role effectively.** Leveraging your love and abilities as parents in the service of fighting an eating disorder is crucial. This is fairly easy to see in the case of anorexia nervosa, where there is seldom any motivation on the part of the adolescent to recover. Without your strength, your child is left to the devices of the disorder and the downward spiral of weight loss and obsessional thoughts about food and calories. However, the same holds true for bulimia nervosa, where the shame of the illness holds your daughter or son captive. When you are able to be a part of the process, the element of shame actually diminishes as you support your child through these dilemmas.

6. **"Getting together" involves the whole family.** It's not just you who are a resource for your child. In fact, your whole family is able to help, in distinct but definite ways. Everyone in the family is affected when a child has an eating disorder. Everyone is worried or angry or both. Your other children see the effects on you and on their sibling. They are often most articulate about how much their brother or sister has been changed by the disorder. They also have clear memories of activities and qualities that are no longer present in their sibling with an eating disorder. Siblings can provide an avenue of support for their sister or brother who is ill, especially when your child may be angry at you for being firm about requirements for attending therapy or setting a limit on a behavior such as throwing up or not eating. They are also excellent sources of distraction and fun, which are needed when someone is fighting an eating disorder.

7. **The therapist is your consultant, not the boss.** In this sense, all therapy with children and adolescents must acknowledge the importance of family relationships. Therapists may be experts in particular areas, but they are not going home with you and do not routinely have to confront the problems in your home—they do not have to eat meals with your family regularly, clean up the bathrooms, and so on. That's what you do as parents. Therapists can help you think through problems and some-

times may even work independently with your child, with your approval, support, and understanding, when needed. But, ultimately, you are the parent and they are advisers to you as you try to navigate the difficult problems that eating disorders present for you, your child, and your family.

So, there is a way you and your family can help your child who is suffering with an eating disorder. It involves, to start with, discarding the notion that you caused the problem. This idea is unproven and will cripple you in your efforts to help. Next, you need to learn all you can about how people with eating disorders think and behave, what motivates them to do what they do. When you do this, you are better prepared to counter them instead of being surprised and taken for a ride. Any therapist you find, regardless of his or her approach, should want to involve you. You should ask about how you will be involved and how you can help. According to some approaches, the therapist sees his or her job as helping you help your child, whereas others that you may find attractive might see you in a more supportive role. In any case, you need to know what the treatment is, what its goals are, and what you will be doing to support it and your child. You should not sit back, but should take responsibility for your child. Don't let an eating disorder "de-skill" you as a parent; don't assume that you no longer know anything. Instead, assume you have a right to know what treatment your child is receiving, a right to look for ways you can help, and a responsibility to ensure that your child is getting the best treatment.

The rest of this book is designed to help you grow more confident in playing an active role in your child's (and your) struggle with an eating disorder. We hope to educate you more about what eating disorders are and how they can affect your child and family. We will review the kinds of treatment options you are likely to find and help you determine how you can be a part of each of these types of treatments. We also will provide you with examples of the kinds of problems you may face and how you might negotiate them. We hope this will help to make you feel more empowered and, with that, even more capable and responsible as, with your help, your son or daughter combats an eating disorder.

FOR MORE INFORMATION

Bruch, H., *Eating Disorders: Obesity, Anorexia Nervosa, and the Person Within*, 1973. New York: Basic Books.

Bruch, H., *The Golden Cage: The Enigma of Anorexia Nervosa*, 1978. Cambridge, MA: Harvard University Press.

Crisp, A., *Anorexia Nervosa: Let Me Be*, 1995. Hove, England: Erlbaum.

Dare, C., and I. Eisler, Family Therapy for Anorexia Nervosa, in D. M. Garner and P. E. Garfinkel, Editors, *Handbook of Treatment for Eating Disorders*, Second Edition, 1997. New York: Guilford Press, pp. 307–324.

Lock, J., D. le Grange, W. S. Agras, and C. Dare, *Treatment Manual for Anorexia Nervosa: A Family-Based Approach*, 2001. New York: Guilford Press.

Minuchin, S., B. Rosman, and I. Baker, *Psychosomatic Families: Anorexia Nervosa in Context*, 1978. Cambridge, MA: Harvard University Press.

CHAPTER 3

DON'T WASTE TIME ON "WHY?"

IS THIS MY FAULT?

Mike woke up at 3:00 in the morning again. His wife, Susan, was already awake. They were worrying about their daughter Anna, who had anorexia. Mike was lamenting the time he had spent talking to his children about the importance of regular exercise. Now Anna wouldn't stop exercising. Susan blamed herself for focusing attention on good nutrition. Now Anna could tell you every food's calorie content and fat grams. Susan was also berating herself for having fashion magazines at home. Now Anna spent an inordinate amount of time looking at herself in the mirror, pinching nonexistent fat on her stomach and thighs. Mike and Susan were sure they had somehow caused Anna's illness. They felt sick with guilt and overwhelmed with doubt about how to proceed.

Perhaps the biggest hurdle you face in trying to figure out how to help your child is the message, both covert and overt, that you must have caused this problem. Something you did as a parent, some failure on your part, some trauma you unconsciously inflicted on your child, resulted in the development of an eating disorder. As we'll discuss, however, the causes of eating disorders remain unknown, and your possible role is at best uncertain. There may be things we do as parents that increase the risk to our children of a variety of problems, both emotional and physical. However, none of those things we might do—for example, worrying about weight, being vegetarians, or eating unhealthily—appear to be specific enough to warrant being labeled a cause of eating disorders.

The truth is that causes of illnesses, especially psychological illnesses, are not easily discoverable. Remember, it took several thousand years to discover the bacterial and viral causes of illnesses like smallpox and pneumonia, and for infectious illnesses the line of causation is direct: Exposure to these bacteria or viruses will ultimately lead to the development of an infectious illness. (Although some attempts have been made to explain anorexia nervosa as a result of exposure to streptococcus, there is no evidence that this is the usual cause of this illness.) An explanation for how psychological illnesses arise, including those with a very clear genetic basis, relies on a much more complex theory of causation that is both indirect and interactive. It is fairly easy to show that by ridding the environment of certain bacteria, pneumonia won't develop. But it's impossible to rid the environment of genetics or vice versa (in fact, they evolve together and inform one another).

Despite the complexity involved in uncovering causation for psychological illnesses, and for eating disorders specifically, theorists have tended to support their recommendations for treatment on the basis of presumed causes. This is confusing and at times misleading. Psychological treatments clearly do not depend on specific knowledge of causation. If they did, we would have little hope of finding helpful interventions. This means that you don't need to understand what has caused your daughter's or son's eating disorder to get help. In fact, dwelling on what may have caused the problem often diverts parents' energies from helping their child. And like Mike and Susan, many parents who get mired in the question "Why?" end up with nowhere to point the finger of blame but at themselves and then become paralyzed by guilt.

Although eating disorders have been around a long time (some contend that there is evidence of eating disorders as far back as ancient Egypt), modern recognition of these illnesses dates from the first descriptions of anorexia nervosa in the late 19th century by Sir William Gull in England and Charles Lasegue in France. Since it was first described, theories about the etiology of anorexia nervosa have ranged from viewing it as a purely physical disease to seeing it as the result of societal forces and not a disease at all. In contrast, bulimia nervosa was first described only in 1979 and was initially seen as "an ominous variant of anorexia nervosa." Bulimia nervosa as a distinct disorder has emerged over the ensuing years. Its cause is also unknown, but it is usually described as having biological, social, and psychological roots.

A CLOSER LOOK AT INDIVIDUAL FACTORS IN CAUSATION

At this point in the evolution of our understanding, eating disorders overall appear to be multifactorial—that is, caused by the interaction of many factors. In the following pages we review some of the factors that theoretically contribute to causing anorexia and bulimia to help you understand (1) how little we actually know about the causes of eating disorders and (2) how assuming we know the cause can lead us down paths of treatment that may not be helpful.

Although it's certainly not a bad thing to have some theoretical ideas about the cause of an illness, when these ideas remain untested but still become gospel for therapists—as has happened for eating disorders, particularly anorexia nervosa—treatments that aren't based on these ideas often remain unexplored as well. And when these ideas center on parents' contribution to cause, they can remove parents as a key ingredient in recovery by disabling them through guilt and creating counterproductive therapist bias against them. The mental health field saw the same thing happen with schizophrenia and autism: The development of these severe psychiatric disorders was typically laid at the parents' doorstep until a deeper understanding of the biological causes of these illnesses was gained. By explaining what we do know about various potential causes for eating disorders in this chapter, we hope to convince you that you are not to blame any more than parents of children with schizophrenia or autism were ever at fault. Putting self-blame behind you will restore your confidence in your ability to help with the problems that eating disorders present for your child. As you're reading about the *theorized* causes of eating disorders, remember that your goal is to go beyond these theories to embrace the need for change and begin to take action.

It's Biology!

There's actually some interesting and important research on the biological and genetic aspects of eating disorders. For example, studies show that anorexia, bulimia, and EDNOS (eating disorder not otherwise specified) all tend to aggregate in families, especially among first-degree female relatives. Eating disorders are three to five times more common in families in which a person is found to have such a disorder, than in families in which no one has had an eating disorder. Still, of course, the vast majority of family members, male and female, do not have an eating disorder. One way researchers have tried to refine these observations about family clustering of eating disorders is by checking to see if identical twins who are raised separately have similar rates of illness. Identical twins have exactly the same genetic makeup (or nearly so), so any differences in the occurrence of eating disorders between identical twins who are raised in different families are likely to be due to the different environmental factors. What investigators have found is that there's a significantly increased risk in twins that appears to be genetic rather than environmental. So, vulnerability to eating disorders appears to be inherited. Because, at least for now, we can't do much about our genes, we can't entirely blame parents, families, or society for the problem.

Not only do eating disorders appear to be heritable, but it's possible that certain personality traits and susceptibility to certain behaviors may also be inherited. Traits such as perfectionism, obsessionality, feeding behaviors, and negative mood states, which are associated with eating disorders, may also be heritable and thereby constitute particular vulnerability for developing eating problems. So far, researchers haven't figured out very much about this, but the idea is that eating disorders are caused indirectly, at least in part, by these inherited personality characteristics. It seems likely that this is true. The problem is that the same characteristics may lead to very healthy outcomes. We've observed this many times. For instance, a young boy with anorexia has a mother who is a CEO and a father who is a doctor. They share many personality traits like perfectionism, drive, and obsessionality, but the outcomes are totally different, because in the parents these traits are applied to work, whereas in the boy they are applied to a preoccupation with dieting and weight.

Other research suggests that certain neurotransmitters are involved in vulnerability toward developing eating disorders. Neurotransmitters are chemicals in the brain that affect a variety of brain functions such as sleep, appetite, mood, and attention. When something goes awry with these chemicals, problems in any of these areas may result. Many neurotransmitters have been implicated in eating disorders (e.g., dopamine, norepinephrine, and serotonin). Probably the most important of the neurotransmitters currently being studied is serotonin. It appears that problems with regulating this brain chemical are related to both anorexia and bulimia. The exact nature of what goes wrong isn't clear, and, unfortunately, medications that aim to fix the problem (and which are effective for depression and anxiety problems) don't work as well with eating disorders. (They do, however, help somewhat with bulimia and may help with *weight-restored* anorexia—when a person's weight has returned to normal but there has been little change in thinking or behavior to ensure that such gains will be preserved.) So, the argument goes that for some reason (inheritance, environmental stress, nutrition) something goes wrong with one or more of these (or other not yet identified) neurotransmitters, which increases the likelihood that an eating disorder will start. Again, this may indeed be true, and medications may someday be of more help in treatment than they are now, but focusing on neurotransmitters alone is unlikely to be enough because the attendant behaviors and thoughts appear to have a life of their own that is reinforced through habit and time. Unless those thought processes and behaviors are addressed directly, targeting neurotransmitters through medications isn't likely to "cure" the disorder.

It's All in the Head!

Dora was 13 when she began restricting her foods in an attempt to lower her weight. She had always been small and thin and did not like the idea of growing bigger. Dora was a bit of a loner. She could socialize with others when she had to, but she clearly preferred to read or study. She showed no romantic interest and shared none of her friends' enthusiasm for boy-girl parties. She was very close to her mother, who had seen Dora from an early age as a shy and vulnerable girl who needed her help to negotiate social challenges.

The early descriptions of anorexia by Gull and Lasegue dovetailed with the emerging psychoanalytic movement in psychiatry and psychology that was to have profound influence on psychiatric treatment for half a century. Psychoanalysis is fundamentally a dyadic (that is, one therapist meeting with one patient) treatment. It also contends that psychological problems stem from early deprivations, traumas, and fantasies related to parents. The approach is basically designed to be used with adult patients (though Sigmund Freud, a famous psychoanalyst, occasionally treated children, and his daughter, Anna Freud, designed treatments for adolescents and children), whose fantasy life is explored through free association and dream interpretation. Patients with anorexia nervosa were seen as reasonable candidates for the psychoanalytic method, and their symptoms of self-starvation were interpreted in various ways. The early theoreticians relied heavily on Freud's understanding of sexual repression as the origin of all mental illness, and as a result, their theories of anorexia coincide with this idea. Thus, early psychoanalytic theory focused on guilt and oral impregnation fantasies, with weight loss seen as a defense mechanism—that is, "not eating" was a way of avoiding sexual thoughts and feelings. Although it has been observed that patients with anorexia are often sexually avoidant and may struggle with interpersonal intimacy, it's not clear whether this is more a result of the disease (starvation, for example, leads to lower sexual hormone levels, and this in turn leads to lowered sexual desire) than the cause.

Later, but still based in the psychoanalytic tradition, Hilde Bruch suggested that the person with anorexia is suffering from an "inadequate sense of self." By this she meant that the patient was socially immature and psychologically underdeveloped. As a result of not feeling confident and assertive, such adolescents turn to other ways of expressing their feelings, especially their anger. Thus, restrictive eating and related disturbed eating patterns are seen as forms of "acting out" the frustration and feelings of inadequacy that these adolescents experience. To assist with these problems, psychoanalytic treatment aims at helping to "find a voice" for this deficient self that substitutes psychological understanding and expression as opposed to disturbed eating as a way of communicating. Indeed, these adolescents often seem immature, naïve, and not particularly assertive as compared with their peers. In fact, the theoretical idea that adolescents with anorexia need help with finding a sense of identity makes a great deal of sense. How to help them best accomplish that task in the context of a serious illness like anorexia is less clear.

It's All in the Family!

Sam's parents did not get along. His father was a busy surgeon, and his mother participated in many charity events and social activities. They seldom had overt conflicts, but they also were seldom together. Sam's father left for work at four thirty in the morning and returned after dinner. Sam's mother was often out in the evening at fund-raising planning meetings. When Sam stopped eating, no one noticed for quite some time. By the time his father finally asked Sam if he was losing weight and arranged for a physical exam, he had lost almost 25 pounds. When the family sat down together for therapy, it was the first time they could remember having been together for several weeks.

Tilly's mother had sent her to live with her father when she was 12 because she and Tilly were fighting all the time. This arrangement went all right until Tilly's father remarried.

Tilly and her stepmother did not get along well. Tilly felt picked on, and her stepmother felt she wasn't respected. Tilly moved back with her mother. During this period, Tilly began to diet and throw up. She said she felt fat and ugly and no one liked her. She had few friends and was very isolated. Her mother was also quite busy with her own work and social life.

When family therapy arrived on the scene in the 1960s and 1970s, it was developed from a psychoanalytic base. Like practitioners of psychoanalysis, many family therapists see anorexia nervosa as a symptom of underlying pathology, this time located in the family as a whole. Therefore, conventional family intervention tries to modify perceived problems within the family or, if this fails, to remove the child from the family. Yet another form of family therapy, so-called structural family therapy for anorexia (probably the best-known approach), was devised based on clinical observations of families by Salvador Minuchin (a pioneer in family therapy for anorexia nervosa). Because the child played a critical role in the family's overall avoidance of conflict, self-starvation was seen as powerfully supported by the family, though its members were not aware of this. Structural family therapy tries to alter family organization by identifying and challenging what are believed to be inappropriate alliances between parents and children, encouraging the development of stronger sibling support of one another, and promoting open communication. The aim is to reduce the child's emotional involvement with parents and to improve the effectiveness of the parents. So this approach also strongly supported the idea that families, and particularly parents, are in some way the cause of anorexia nervosa and without help will only perpetuate the problem. Data about the idea that families of patients are truly "pathological" are surprisingly conflicting. Some studies suggest that these families do have unique problems of the type that Minuchin described, whereas others don't appear to detect differences between these families and so-called normal families. Even if there are such differences, though, it isn't clear how they relate to the development of an eating disorder. In other words, a family can have many problems (as in Tilly's case), but the direct link between such problems and their causing an eating disorder is a *leap* that cannot and really should not be made.

It's a Stage. She'll Outgrow It!

Mimi has always been a good student, but "slow to warm" socially. When her family moved to another city at the beginning of sixth grade, it was not very surprising that she struggled to make new friends. She complained about the new school and about being lonely. She fantasized about going back to her own town, where she was happier and felt more accepted. Just after the winter holiday, Mimi had her first menstrual period. She told her mother that it hurt and she didn't like it. Although her mother tried to be supportive, Mimi remained very upset. Not long afterward, Mimi began to diet. She told her mother that she had an upset stomach or was too nervous to eat. Over time she ate less and less, and her parents became increasingly concerned. When the gym teacher called to ask Mimi's parents to meet with her about Mimi's weight, they were not surprised, but they didn't know what to do either.

Eating disorders generally begin during adolescence. This is a principal reason why many theorists have viewed the disorders as related to issues of this developmental period, specifically with struggles for autonomy. A model for the cause of anorexia was developed by Arthur Crisp, a London psychiatrist, who speculated in the 1970s and 1980s that anorexia was the result of phobic avoidance of adolescence. That is, Crisp suggested that adolescents who develop anorexia were anxious about the physical changes associated with puberty, about establishing a more socially independent identity, and about entering social relations as sexually mature beings. The weight loss that resulted from excessive dieting and exercise restored the body shape and hormonal status of preadolescence, and the medical and psychological secondary effects returned the adolescent to the more dependent status of a younger child. Therefore, the child apparently accomplished her goal of avoiding adolescent struggles. This theory, which is said to apply to adolescents with either anorexia or bulimia, shows a healthy respect for the normal processes of adolescents and families and provides a very good context for thinking about therapy for teenagers. Still, it is unclear how best to employ the insight that developmental issues are key to understanding eating disorders. And in a certain sense the theory raises the question of causation: After all, the developmental challenges associated with adolescence are common to everyone, so why do only some teenagers develop eating disorders in response? No one knows for sure.

It's Hollywood!

> Tom spent hours studying himself in the mirror. He compared himself with the male models and athletes he saw in magazines. He felt his arms were too flabby and undefined. He wanted to be "cut" and lean. He wanted a "six-pack" of abdominal muscles. He began with lifting weights and cutting down on desserts and fast foods, but soon he was counting calories and throwing up to make sure he would lose weight. His friends noticed that he was looking very muscular and trim. Several girls talked to him and flirted. Tom was sure he was on the right track.

A third approach to the cause of eating disorders focuses on the social and cultural forces on developing adolescents that may lead to increased problems with eating behaviors, body image concerns, and poor self-esteem. Although these forces have been influencing adolescent girls for some time, it's pretty clear that the same forces are acting on boys more than they used to. There are several forces that are considered likely culprits: media images, Western cultural ideals, and wealth.

Media

The forces imposed by the media influence children fairly early. For girls, Barbie dolls and similar toys set very early standards for unrealistic expectations in regard to body shape and size. For boys, male images of unrealistic body mass and musculature are increasing as well. When the Han Solo action figure based on the *Star Wars* movies first came out in the 1970s, he had human proportions, but the more recent action figure is unrealistically muscled. In addition, studies of *Playboy* and *Playgirl* centerfolds document a continuing trend toward ever-decreasing body fat and greater leanness in the male and female models represented. Even a cursory look at a fashion magazine or television program discerns a host of examples of very thin women and men with extremely lean and muscular bodies modeling the latest styles. The basic difficulty is that these toys, images, and models set an unhealthy standard for beauty that vulnerable children and young adolescent males and females then aspire to.

> Lia wanted to be a model when she grew up. She bought all the fashion magazines she could find. She shopped at every opportunity and spent a lot of time getting dressed for school and outings. During her second year of high school, Lia went to a modeling agency. She was told that she had a good face but she needed to lose 15 pounds if she wanted to be considered. Lia was not overweight, but she decided that becoming a model would be worth losing those pounds. Lia began dieting, exercising, and taking diet pills to curb her appetite and laxatives to "cleanse" her system. She lost about 8 pounds, and her friends and family said she looked great. However, Lia felt she could be thinner. She continued to restrict her intake, but when she did eat, even a normal meal, she would throw it up.

Western Cultural Ideals of Beauty

That the popular media have a great influence on all of our lives, especially the lives of adolescents, is obvious. Social values in regard to food and weight have long influenced our behavior. In the 16th century, for example, overweight was in, which made eating in abundance desirable, whereas being unduly thin was a mark of social inferiority and even sickness. In the Pacific islands of Tonga, eating disorders were unknown and overeating and corpulence were considered desirable until television was introduced in the early 1990s, after which eating disorders started to appear and young girls and women began to worry about their weight and to diet.

Western ideas of beauty and body shape are permeating other cultures all over the world, particularly in Asia. In the last several years, eating disorders have apparently been developing rapidly in Japan, Taiwan, Singapore, and Hong Kong. Studies of immigrants suggest that young women who move from a non-Western culture to a Western culture are at increased risk for eating disturbances.

Indira's parents, both engineers, moved to the United States from India when she was about 2 years old. Indira had done very well in school, excelling in both academics and athletics. However, at the beginning of high school, Indira began to lose weight and to complain about her skin color. She asked her parents for blue-tinted contact lenses. Indira explained her desire to lose weight and wear blue contact lenses as a way to fit in better with her mostly white friends in the private school she attended. Her parents were concerned about Indira's developing identity and saw her anorexia nervosa as a manifestation of her conflicts about being a minority person in a white majority group.

Indira's description of her experience is in line with some cross-cultural studies suggesting that immigrants, especially non-white immigrants, are experiencing increasing problems with eating disorders. The notion is that among these adolescents there is increased cultural strain, that is, an increased need to "fit in" and be "acceptable" relative to the white cultural thin ideal. To accomplish this, some teenagers try to change their appearance, particularly their weight, to become more desirable and to compete more successfully. Becoming psychologically and emotionally invested in meeting Western standards of beauty regarding thinness causes some of these young people to pursue unhealthy weight loss strategies to the point where they develop eating disorders.

Related to the problems inherent in the Western idea of beauty are feminist perspectives on eating disorders and their development. The basic idea is that Western ideas of beauty, in their focus on thin body ideals, are part of a large cultural attack on women and women's bodies that is designed to keep women disempowered. This is accomplished by setting unrealistic standards of attractiveness. When women feel that they don't meet these standards, the result is low self-esteem, poor self-worth, and less ability to perform in the culture. In addition, of course, these feelings and perceptions lead to eating disorders—an effect of this larger attack on women.

The feminist perspective on the development of eating disorders is instructive in several ways. First, it integrates the ideas of beauty, power, and gender, which are common themes in eating-disordered patients. It also synthesizes the roles of culture and media in the development of eating problems. Further, it suggests that even women in the wealthier classes (see the next section) are not immune. Although not usually articulated, the feminist perspective also provides a partial rationale for why and how eating disorders might be more common among gay men. However, it has less to say about eating disorders among heterosexual men, athletes, and religious persons, who are less likely to be victims of media and other mainstream social forces identified in the feminist literature in the same way.

Wealth

Eating disorders, especially anorexia, have long been associated with higher socioeconomic status. The maxim "You can never be too rich or too thin" captures the essence of this association. There are several possible origins of this relationship. The first is rather concrete: The wealthy no longer have to worry about basic survival, and being thin manifests this. The second is more subtle, that is, that wealth confers a special status—a superior status—such that one doesn't need to eat. Of course, the confluence of wealth and fashion fuels the fantasy that to be rich is to be thin and vice versa. In fact, it appears that anorexia does seem to cluster more commonly among wealthier families. This is not to say it doesn't occur in the less wealthy, because it certainly does.

However, it is less clear that wealth itself is the risk factor. It may be that some families are wealthier in part, as we have suggested earlier, because of some temperamental or personality traits that when applied to business lead to work and success, but when applied to dieting lead to anorexia. Thus, it may be a tautology to see wealth per se as the cause of anorexia. On the other hand, other eating disorders such as bulimia and related syndromes don't appear to cluster to the same extent according to socioeconomic status. Instead, they are more widely distributed socioeconomically, culturally, and racially. Yet it may be that patients with bulimia are more sensitive to the influences of culture, media, or status (wealth), and this sensitivity may contribute to the development or maintenance of their eating-disordered behaviors, but how much or how specifically is speculative.

It's Due to Trauma!

There is a long-standing association between mental illness in general and sexual abuse and trauma. Researchers have been particularly interested in sexual abuse and eating disorders because many young women with eating disorders reported experiences of this kind to their doctors or therapists. Most studies have found that sexual or physical abuse is, in fact, a risk factor for eating problems, particularly bulimia, but no specific link between eating disorders and abuse has been established. The basic theory is that sexual trauma may heighten anxieties about the body, exacerbating an already exaggerated emphasis on weight and shape and leading to the development of eating-disordered thoughts and behaviors. Although certainly reasonable, this theory is not applicable to everyone, inasmuch as most people with eating disorders have not been abused or traumatized. And just as with targeting neurotransmitters, focusing solely on abuse or trauma seems unlikely to alleviate eating disorder symptoms, which take on a "life of their own" over time and need to be addressed specifically. The dilemma for therapists seems to be that it's easy to make sexual abuse or other trauma the sole focus of treatment because abuse is such a devastating event, yet doing so, in our opinion, might make it more difficult to treat the eating disorder.

DON'T GET STUCK ON "WHY?"

If it now seems that all of the reasons proposed for the development of an eating disorder make sense—or that none of them do—rest assured that both these statements are true. It's a matter of perspective. It is also true that focusing on why your child has

developed an eating disorder or maintains one may not be very
helpful. Imagine your child does not have anorexia or bulimia
but cancer. No one knows exactly why she developed cancer,
and the treatment prescribed does not aim at the cause of the
cancer but instead targets the effects—removal of the malignancy
and treatment with radiation and chemotherapy to prevent the
growth of new cancerous lesions. Treatment for many childhood
cancers is remarkably effective, even though the cause is often
unknown and the treatment doesn't necessarily aim for it. For
many of the diseases we treat in medicine, this is also the case.
With diabetes, for example, we often don't really know why the
body stops making adequate insulin, but we can control the disease with medications. Another example includes some types of
seizures. We can generally identify the part of the brain in which
the electrical impulses have gone awry, and sometimes we can
perform surgery to resect that part, but usually, more conserva-
tively but just as effectively, we treat the disorder with medications and the seizures are controlled. The list could go on. The
point is that for most illnesses we have to treat symptoms—and in
many cases end up doing away with the disease in the process—
but for mental illnesses we expect treatment to focus on eradicat-
ing the cause. This is largely because psychological and psychiatric research has been so interested in psychological explanations
and conflicts, and this applies particularly to eating disorders. As
we've seen, though, we seldom *know* what the cause is. How can
we hope to eradicate the illness if we treat it by trying to eliminate what we can only guess is the cause?

It's understandable for you to want to know why your child has
developed an eating disorder. It seems a random and unfair event,
causing worry, hazard, and difficulty for your child and family. It's
also understandable that psychologists and psychiatrists find investigating cause fascinating. Unfortunately, although research
into why eating disorders occur may eventually help us prevent
them from developing, we think the subject of cause just lures
practitioners off course. Dwelling on cause in treatment keeps
therapists and parents from dedicating their efforts to the problem at hand—keeping the starving teenager before them alive and
restoring her to health. With your child starving or throwing up in
front of you, a discussion of her genetic vulnerability for anxiety

and eating problems, how controlling you were as parents, how immature she is psychologically, and the problems of society's standards for beauty will likely be distracting and probably take you off track, at least initially. This is time you may not be able to afford to waste. In fact, such meditations and preoccupations sometimes play directly into the hands of the eating disorder by allowing the behaviors and thoughts to persist without confrontation and redirection, for longer periods and with more success. (More on this phenomenon is in Chapter 5.) We know that the longer a person loses weight, maintains low weight, purges, and binges (in other words, the more chronically ill she is), the less likely we will be successful in getting rid of the eating disorder. This is true for any illness. The longer you have diabetes before you are treated, the more difficult it is to control and the more problematic are the long-term effects. The same is true for cancer, heart disease, and other debilitating illnesses. That being the case, it's important to take action quickly and decisively rather than just ponder why.

Setting aside the question of "why?" may be easier said than done. We would prefer the question be deferred or bracketed while the disordered eating behaviors and weight problems remain unresolved. We see these problems as leading to a kind of thinking that is similar to trying to do therapy with someone who is inebriated: You just can't do it, because that person can't process what you're saying. You've got to wait until she is sober, or at least somewhat sober, before you can hope to communicate with her. In the meantime, though, you have to get her sober. That means getting the alcohol out of her system and trying to keep her from drinking again. With eating disorders, at least at the beginning, we think you have to do the same thing. Stop the behaviors that are leading to the problem and keep them from recurring long enough that discussions about the problems associated with the disorder can be approached.

Perhaps the most important reason not to get stuck on "why?" is that your child needs your help. By setting the problem of "why?" to the side, we hope that you will feel less ashamed and guilty, see yourself as an excellent candidate to help your child get the treatment and support he or she needs, and involve yourself in that treatment with confidence and commitment.

FOR MORE INFORMATION

Anderson-Fye, E. P., and A. E. Becker, Sociocultural Aspects of Eating Disorders, in J. K. Thompson, Editor, *Handbook of Eating Disorders and Obesity*, 2004. Hoboken, NJ: Wiley, pp. 565–589.

Bulik, C. M., Genetic and Biological Risk Factors, in J. K. Thompson, Editor, *Handbook of Eating Disorders and Obesity*, 2004. Hoboken, NJ: Wiley, pp. 3–16.

Field, A., Risk Factors for Eating Disorders: An Evaluation of the Evidence, in J. K. Thompson, Editor, *Handbook of Eating Disorders and Obesity*, 2004. Hoboken, NJ: Wiley, pp. 17–32.

Levine, M., and K. Harrison, Media's Role in the Perpetuation and Prevention of Negative Body Image and Disordered Eating, in J. K. Thompson, Editor, *Handbook of Eating Disorders and Obesity*, 2004. Hoboken, NJ: Wiley, pp. 695–717.

Nasser, M., *Culture and Weight Consciousness*, 1997. London: Routledge.

Nasser, M., M. Katzman, and R. Gordon, Editors, *Eating Disorders and Cultures in Transition*, 2001. New York: Brunner-Routledge.

Vandereycken, W., Families of Patients with Eating Disorders, in C. G. Fairburn and K. D. Brownell, Editors, *Eating Disorders and Obesity: A Comprehensive Handbook*, Second Edition, 2002. New York: Guilford Press, pp. 215–220.

Wonderlich, S., Personality and Eating Disorders, in C. G. Fairburn and K. D. Brownell, Editors, *Eating Disorders and Obesity: A Comprehensive Handbook*, Second Edition, 2002. New York: Guilford Press, pp. 204–209.

Wonderlich, S., R. Crosby, J. Mitchell, J. Thompson, J. Redlin, G. Demuth, J. Smyth, and B. Haseltine, Eating Disturbance and Sexual Trauma in Childhood and Adulthood, *International Journal of Eating Disorders*, 2001, *30*, pp. 401–412.

PART II

Understanding Eating Disorders

CHAPTER 4

KNOW WHAT YOU'RE DEALING WITH

The Complexity of Eating Disorders

We probably don't have to tell you that you can't solve a problem unless you know what you're dealing with. Every day, at home and at work, you take steps to figure out what you're up against before devising a strategy for attacking a particular challenge. Whether it's getting the car to run or your checkbook to balance, getting your assistant to be more productive or your sales force to exceed last year's gross, you decide on a solution based on your understanding of the problem. Helping your child overcome an eating disorder is no different.

As you now know, having read Part I of this book, eating disorders are enigmatic and idiosyncratic. There are lots of gaps in our scientific understanding of anorexia and bulimia. What we do know sets eating disorders apart from other psychiatric problems affecting children and adolescents, which has made treating them an ongoing challenge. The gaps in our understanding of these disorders stem from the fact that there is a comparative dearth of research on eating disorders in children and adolescents. For instance, as of the writing of this book, only five published psychological treatment studies have been conducted for anorexia and none for bulimia. To heighten our challenge in the treatment of eating disorders, myths and misconceptions about these disorders abound in the popular media.

It's essential that you know what you're dealing with if you're to help a child who has an eating disorder. In this chapter we give you up-to-date, scientifically based information on anorexia and bulimia. With this foundation, your quest to help your child will gain the greatest possible chance for success.

We can't state this too often: Know the facts. It could save your child's life.

EATING DISORDERS ARE PSYCHOLOGICAL ILLNESSES WITH SERIOUS MEDICAL CONSEQUENCES

Talk about complicated: No other psychological illnesses affecting children and adolescents involve pathological thoughts, behaviors, and emotions that lead to such serious short- and long-term medical complications. Because these disturbances in the way individuals think, feel, and act, in turn, bring about a dramatic change in food consumption, eating disorders can cause physical illness perhaps more than any other mental illness currently known. This means that parents and health care providers must not only understand the psychological workings of these disorders and apply psychological treatments, but must also be alert to what's happening to the child's physical health. In fact, it is fair to say that in most cases you should deal first and foremost with your child's medical status. Starvation poses several medical risks, as we elaborate on in the following pages. Moreover, many of the psychological symptoms you may have noted in your child are the direct consequence of these medical problems. Therefore, it is of paramount importance that your child enter a treatment regimen, whether outpatient, inpatient, or residential, that will attend to her medical status and provide a supportive environment in which the psychological workings of her disorder can begin to be explored.

How Are Eating Disorders Defined?

Eating disorders, as we explained in Chapter 1, are of three main types: anorexia nervosa, bulimia nervosa, and eating disorder not otherwise specified (EDNOS). There are differences between them, but they also share many features. We have to consider both the similarities and the differences when we ask the question, "What is an eating disorder?" It's sometimes difficult to know at the outset which of the three eating disorder diagnoses will be the most accurate, because over time as many as one-third to one-half of patients can eventually be diagnosed with two or more of the different types of eating disorders. Although we mentioned the specific challenges of making an accurate diagnosis of an eating disorder in children and adolescents in Chapter 1, it's important to revisit these issues with an emphasis on helping you identify the overlapping as well as distinguishing characteristics of the particular disorder type.

> Annette, now 16, has been ill with an eating disorder since she was 12 years old. She has spent most of the past 4 years in and out of the hospital. As a result, it has been very hard for her to spend significant periods of time at home with her parents and siblings, to make and keep friends at school, and to have an opportunity to build and learn from meaningful relationships outside her family. In addition, she has fallen seriously behind in her schoolwork even though the hospital unit to which she is usually admitted provides schooling for the adolescents in its program.
>
> Every time Annette is admitted, she is severely emaciated, which requires her doctors to put her on strict bed rest with frequent visits by the nursing and medical staff. Eventually, her weight begins to approach healthy levels again and she is prepared to be discharged to her parents' care. At this time, however, her parents are always told to "back off" as Annette should now take care of her own eating. Unfortunately, every time she tries to eat on her own, she promptly runs to the bathroom to induce vomiting because she "cannot stand" feeling so "full."

The nurses in the hospital would have prevented Annette from vomiting, but at home, following the doctor's advice, her parents are backing off. Consequently, Annette's weight, time and again, spirals downward as she checks in every week with her outpatient pediatrician. Her pediatrician is concerned with the speed at which Annette always manages to lose weight once she is discharged, and he is also very worried because her daily vomiting after every meal has caused her electrolyte levels to drop well within dangerous levels. Every couple of weeks, Annette gets herself admitted to a medical ward to restore her electrolytes to normal levels. Although this is a life-saving necessity, it again takes Annette away from her home environment, her friends, and school. This cycle—going to an eating disorder inpatient unit, back home, and then in and out of the medical unit—as well as receiving a multitude of different medications, has been a sad routine for Annette and her family for many years now.

According to the *Diagnostic and Statistical Manual of Mental Disorders* (the DSM) anorexia nervosa results from the refusal to maintain (or reach, during a period of growth) a weight of 85% of what would be expected for someone of similar height. This is accompanied by an overriding fear of weight gain and a lack of recognition of the physical changes that result from malnutrition. In addition, there is body image distortion (seeing the body as fat when it is actually thin) or denial of the seriousness of the consequences of starvation (for example, not believing heart rates as low as 40 beats per minute are life threatening). For women and adolescent girls, these behaviors and beliefs are accompanied by loss of three consecutive menstrual cycles.

Some people with anorexia nervosa use only extreme dieting techniques by limiting their intake (called the *restricting subtype*), and others engage in binge eating and purging (use of vomiting, laxatives, other purgatives) behaviors (called the *binge/purge subtype*). As we pointed out in Chapter 1, these criteria are most appropriate for adults with anorexia. But among the diagnostic criteria for anorexia, there is the suggestion that failure to grow, an event specific to childhood and adolescence, will substitute for meeting the usual weight-loss criteria. The missing of three consecutive menstrual periods is also an unnecessary criterion if the adolescent has not previously menstruated.

Bulimia nervosa is also defined as having both behavioral and psychological components. Behavioral components include intermittent severe dieting strategies that lead to weight fluctuations while the person maintains an overall weight within the normal range. These dieting strategies are interrupted by episodes of binge eating and compensatory purgative behaviors (purging, exercise, laxative use, etc.). To meet the definition, these types of behaviors must be present for a period of 3 months with an intensity, on average, of at least two episodes a week of binge eating or purging. In addition, for someone to be diagnosed with bulimia nervosa these behaviors should be accompanied by extreme beliefs and attitudes that overemphasize control of shape and weight as the sole or major way to maintain self-worth and self-esteem. Again, these criteria are perhaps most appropriate for adult cases. Children and adolescents developing bulimia may not necessarily meet these frequency criteria (the number of binges and purges per week), as the illness is not so well established yet.

A diagnosis of eating disorder not otherwise specified (EDNOS), however, allows for a considerable range of symptoms and attitudes resulting from some form of abnormal eating or dieting practice and often includes adolescents who don't meet the full criteria for either anorexia or bulimia outlined earlier. What is critical for a diagnosis of EDNOS is that the problem be related to eating, include both behavioral and psychological components, and be severe enough to cause problems. As a consequence of the failure of the current DSM to capture early development of serious eating disorders, children and adolescents often best fall into the category of EDNOS when strict definitions of anorexia and bulimia are used.

If you're a little confused about all this right now, you're not alone. Professionals in our field are still wrestling with just how these three eating disorders are distinct from one another or the degree to which they overlap. What we find helpful, as we said in

Chapter 1, is to take a broader view of eating disorders and look for what is common to anorexia, bulimia, and EDNOS, rather than focus on how they are different.

Medical Complications of Anorexia Nervosa

In Chapter 2 we exhorted you to view yourselves as part of the solution to your child's eating disorder—advice that's difficult to take when your son or daughter is treating you as if you're crazy at best, his or her enemy at worst. In truth, living with a child who has developed anorexia can make you feel as if you *are* insane. The illness is publicly quite visible—the fact that your child is emaciated is plain for all to see (if he or she hasn't shrouded him- or herself in baggy clothing to hide the skeletal frame that you have been pointing to), yet he or she very likely will insist that nothing is wrong. This view of an illness as non-problematic or "perfectly normal" makes anorexia a disorder that we call *ego-syntonic*. The anorexic adolescent may very well view his or her illness with a sense of pride or achievement and protect the illness through denial. As a consequence, your child may not willingly seek or accept treatment. In fact, this peculiar characteristic of anorexia tends to make your job as a parent more difficult overall when it comes to the medical complications of the illness. Adolescents without anorexia may notice a particular physical ailment, such as stomach pain or a headache, and be more than likely to bring that knowledge or awareness to their parents' attention. Adolescents with anorexia, however, will almost certainly not appreciate the potential seriousness of any of their symptoms and, consequently, will not bring up the issue with you, their parents. Likewise, if you should note anything that worries you about your adolescent's health, you will experience the uphill and frustrating battle of trying to convince your adolescent that something serious might be wrong and that there is a need to check with your family pediatrician.

Let's say that you're Linda's mother. Linda is 17 and has always been slender. You weren't particularly concerned about this; after all, she appears to be happy, does well at school, and seems to get along with her friends. All the women in your family have been "slow starters" in regard to the onset of menses, and you haven't been very concerned about the fact that Linda has never had a period at age 17. Your concerns were also brushed aside a year ago when you took Linda for a visit with her pediatrician and the doctor said not to worry and put Linda on the birth control pill. The reasoning behind the doctor's intervention was that the medication would start her period and thus "take care of things." In the last year, though, you have noticed that Linda has become increasingly withdrawn, even looking depressed at times. She remains picky about her food and doesn't eat as much as you think she should, and you've begun to wonder whether her frequent running doesn't perhaps make things worse. You decide to ignore your pediatrician's words of comfort and take Linda to see someone who specializes in eating disorders.

After you, your spouse, and Linda have talked to a team of specialists, you all learn that Linda's health has been compromised to a much greater extent than anyone has imagined. It turns out that she meets the criteria for anorexia. In addition to your worries about her mood and the fact that she's much more isolated socially and not as confident as you thought your 17-year-old would be, Linda's physical symptoms have alarmed the specialty team greatly. The medical examination revealed that in addition to Linda's low weight, which has persisted for several years now, she suffers from osteoporosis (a condition of brittle bones that fracture easily, which is quite common in postmenopausal females but very uncommon in someone who is healthy and of Linda's age). Making things worse, it turns out that Linda is no longer 67 inches tall as her medical records have always confirmed. Now she has lost a full inch in height (losing height is, again, quite common in older females who suffer from osteoporosis, but highly unlikely in someone as young as Linda). You learn from the psychiatric team that treatment for Linda is going to be very complex, for it will not only address her weight loss, which is something she dreads, but will also help her with mood and social isolation. At the same time, the medical part of the treatment team will have to address the lack of menses (being maintained artificially by the birth control pill) and figure out how best to make sure that further loss in bone density can be prevented.

There's no denying that all of these health problems are disturbing, especially when the child herself is denying there's anything wrong. Parents can get so caught up in the battle over eating, however, that some miss the early signs that life-threatening starvation has begun. Once the adolescent has reached an obvious state of emaciation, one of the first telling signs that starvation has reached serious proportions is the loss of menstruation, in postmenarcheal girls and women, as body fat declines. What can be confusing is that, for some, amenorrhea sets in after relatively little weight loss, but for others, only very low weight triggers the loss of periods. Because the process of loss of menses seems to vary considerably from adolescent to adolescent, some have argued that amenorrhea should no longer be required to make a diagnosis of anorexia. As noted earlier, this may be especially true for adolescents who do not have firmly established menstrual cycles. For obvious reasons, it also becomes a confusing issue in the case of boys with an eating disorder, as there is no clear equivalent to loss of menses. If you're worried about a son who may have an eating disorder, you'll have to be alert to the signs of other medical complications.

In addition to causing loss of menses, severe malnutrition usually leads to a variety of serious medical consequences. Several systems are impacted by self-starvation: the central nervous system and the cardiovascular, renal, hematologic, gastrointestinal, metabolic, and endocrine systems. The most significant acute problems are bradycardia, hypothermia, and dehydration. All of these complications can become life threatening. The most important chronic medical problems for adolescents with anorexia are the potential for significant growth retardation (your adolescent with anorexia may not maximize her growth spurt and may consequently fail to achieve optimal height); pubertal delay or interruption, which can have serious consequences in terms of menses and fertility; and peak bone mass reduction, which can lead to osteoporosis or osteopenia (an increased porosity of the bone associated with frequent fractures). In addition, many other side effects of malnutrition are often noted:

1. **Hypothermia:** Lower than normal body temperature. You may notice that your adolescent wears extra layers of clothing to try to stay warm even when it is warm outside.

2. **Hypotension:** Decreased blood pressure (a systolic blood pressure of less than 90 millimeters of mercury for adults). Low blood pressure generally has no clinical symptoms, so you might not notice that anything is amiss with your child. However, if it is associated with decreased tissue perfusion (e.g., poor circulation causing cold hands and feet, or slow healing of cuts), your child may have increased heart rate, sweating, lightheadedness, and pallor. This is called *shock*, and it is deadly.

3. **Bradycardia:** Decreased heart rate (for adults, fewer than 60 beats per minute) or a slow pulse. In someone with anorexia, this correlates with the severity of the illness but can be seen only by taking a pulse or performing an electrocardiogram.

4. **Changes in skin and hair texture:** Skin becomes dry and flaky, and hair becomes brittle and can thin out quite dramatically. This is perhaps one of the few consequences of starvation that you, as a parent, may begin to notice.

5. **Lanugo:** There is often a development of fine, downy body hair, most noticeable on your adolescent's face and the back of her neck. This is another way in which the body is attempting to accommodate to the slowdown in metabolism, essentially trying to maintain core body temperature. As with the other skin and hair changes, you might actually notice this growth of fine hair on your child's face or neck.

6. **Growth hormone changes:** There is often an increase in growth hormone secretion, which can be detected only through laboratory tests.

7. **Hypothalamic hypogonadism:** This describes a decrease in sex hormones, which causes an absence of menses and leads to infertility. Blood tests can reveal this condition.

8. **Bone marrow hypoplasia:** Decreased blood cell production, including a low count of red blood cells, white blood cells, and platelets, which leads to anemia. The anemia may contribute to your noticing your child being a bit more fatigued than usual. The lowered white cell counts have not been found to be associated with decreased immune functioning in the case of anorexia.

9. **Structural abnormalities of the brain, generalized atrophy of the brain, and occasional regional atrophy:** This describes a decreased size of the brain or parts of the brain. There are no clear clinical signs of this happening in your child; it can be detected only if you specifically request a neuropsychological evaluation.

10. **Additional changes in electrical brain activity:** The electroencephalograms (EEGs, which show brain activity with electrodes placed on the head) of children with anorexia are often abnormal. You will not be able to see these abnormalities just by looking at your child.

11. **Cardiac dysfunction:** This may include peripheral edema, decreased cardiac diameter, narrowed left ventricular wall, decreased response to exercise demand, pericardial effusion, and superior mesenteric artery syndrome. Your adolescent may describe fatigue, decreased ability to exert him- or herself, and a swelling of his or her legs. Cardiac complications are often lethal and can be confirmed only with the help of an electrocardiogram.

12. **Gastrointestinal difficulties:** Delayed gastric emptying, gastric dilatation, or decreased intestinal lipase and lactase, for example, may manifest itself in your child as abdominal discomfort; your child may complain about a sense of stomach fullness after eating very little. Again, only sophisticated tests will help you confirm the true nature of your child's gastrointestinal problems.

Although these complications are most typical for adolescents with anorexia, restricting subtype, several other complications that are related to binge-eating and purging behaviors in particular should also be considered. These complications will be clearer once we've discussed the medical issues associated with bulimia nervosa.

Medical Complications of Bulimia Nervosa

Nora, now 17, had been binge eating and purging since she was 15 years old. Over the past several months, as she neared her graduation, she felt increasing pressure to excel in school. Unfortunately, she was also being pressured by her boyfriend to become sexually intimate, something she was afraid to do because she was ashamed of her "thunder thighs" and her "fat stomach." She began to purge more frequently, resulting in blood appearing in her vomitus. She was increasingly dizzy when she stood up, and her heart would race. One afternoon, as she went to her car from school, she fainted. Her friends called 911, and she was taken to the emergency room, where she was found to be dehydrated and anemic; she also had a low potassium level.

Bulimia is a more secretive illness than anorexia, making it easier for your adolescent to hide her symptoms. The medical complications are also not as evident as might be the case with anorexia, for most adolescents with bulimia usually have a healthy appearance. In contrast to anorexia, bulimia is described as "ego-alien," which implies that the sufferer is embarrassed or ashamed about her symptoms and is therefore hesitant to seek treatment.

Children and teenagers with bulimia nervosa rarely approach the low weights associated with anorexia. In fact, although some patients with bulimia are quite underweight and others quite overweight, most fall within normal weight limits. Unfortunately, we don't have much research data on teenagers with bulimia. We do, however, know that doctors who see such cases find the same signs and symptoms that are typical of adults with bulimia. We can then assume that the medical complications of bulimia will be about the same for your teenage daughter or son as for adult patients. We don't have any mortality figures for bulimia in either adults or teenagers, but certainly the medical complications that sometimes require hospitalization—hypokalemia, esophageal tears, gastric disturbances, dehydration, and orthostatic blood pressure changes—can result in death. There are indeed case examples of adults with bulimia nervosa who died because of esophageal tears, with extensive internal bleeding. Because many teenagers with bulimia nervosa have periods of starvation similar to those of teenagers with anorexia, many medical complications of bulimia are the same as those of anorexia. However, because bulimia nervosa is mostly characterized by binge-eating and purging episodes, there are some unique medical complications that are more common in bulimia. These are:

1. **Hypokalemic alkalosis or acidosis:** Low potassium level (less than 3.5 milliequivalents per liter in adults) and acid/base imbalance go hand in hand, because changes in the acid/base balance affect the functional potassium levels. With low potassium, you may notice general weakness and malaise in your child. The most catastrophic effect of a low potassium level, however, may be abnormal electrical conduction in the heart, which can lead to death.

2. **Hypochloremia:** This describes low serum chloride levels resulting from the body's attempt to retain electroneutrality in the presence of an acid/base imbalance. The lack of chloride increases serum bicarbonate levels, which then leads to metabolic alkalosis. What this means is that the body has accumulated too much of an alkaline substance (e.g., bicarbonate) and does not have enough acid to effectively neutralize the effects of the alkali. This can be detected only with blood tests.

3. **Dehydration:** Because of decreased body fluid, your child may have dry skin and complain of fatigue or lightheadedness upon standing.

4. **Renal problems:** These can include prerenal azotemia, acute and chronic renal failure. *Azotemia* describes increased nitrogenous wastes in the blood (urea and creatinine), which are a sign of kidney dysfunction. Azotemia may be associated with generalized fatigue, paleness, anorexia (loss of appetite), and swelling. *Prerenal* indicates that the cause for this is not within but before the kidney, such as reduced fluid volume associated with the dehydration of eating disorders. *Acute and chronic renal failure* describes kidney malfunction or failure.

5. **Seizures:** Seizures are abnormal, sudden, excessive discharges of brain neurons. During a generalized seizure, the type of seizure generally relevant here, your child may experience a loss of consciousness, muscle jerking, tongue biting, and urinary incontinence.

6. **Cardiac arrhythmias:** These are irregular heartbeats.

Many adolescents with arrhythmias don't have any clinical signs or symptoms, although in some he or she might notice palpitations (most commonly), shortness of breath, chest pain, lightheadedness, and loss of consciousness. Arrhythmias can be lethal.

7. **Myocardial toxicity caused by emetine** (using ipecac syrup to purge): Cardiac muscle poisoning by ipecac may cause cardiomyopathy, which may manifest itself in your child as loss of consciousness, fatigue, and arrhythmia. It too can be lethal.

8. **Enamel loss and multiple caries:** As a result of the tooth damage often caused by bulimia, your child may report frequent toothaches, or you may notice that the general status of her dental health (and appearance) has deteriorated. In cases of frequent vomiting over time, some patients have lost almost all their teeth.

9. **Swollen parotid glands, elevated serum amylase levels, and gastric distention:** Your child with swollen parotid glands may look as if she has "chipmunk cheeks."

10. **Cramps and tetany:** Tetany describes intermittent paroxysmal muscle spasms. Tetany may also be associated with nervousness, numbness, and tingling of the arms and legs.

A vital aspect in the care of eating-disordered patients is an appreciation for the medical complications of such illnesses. It is often too easy for both parents and clinicians to underestimate the severity of these illnesses. It is only when a comprehensive evaluation of the adolescent's medical status has been completed and medical follow-up has been established that the psychiatrist or psychologist can focus on appropriate treatment to address the eating disorder symptoms and the concomitant psychosocial issues. So, always make 100% sure that your child has received a thorough medical workup by a pediatrician who understands eating disorders. In addition, make sure you're present for much of this examination so you can add information that the physician needs to reach a complete understanding of your child's medical status. Too often we find that the illness, whether it's anorexia or bulimia, prevents the teenager from sharing all the vital facts with the doctor.

EATING DISORDERS ARE OFTEN ACCOMPANIED BY OTHER PSYCHOLOGICAL ILLNESSES

It's not uncommon for eating disorders to be accompanied by other types of mental illness, at least in adults. We have less information in this area regarding teenagers, but you should be aware of this possibility. Other disorders that occur at the same time as the eating disorder—a condition referred to as *comorbidity*—can complicate your child's treatment and possibly reduce the success of treatment if the comorbid illness(es) isn't managed well.

Miranda was first brought in for treatment when she was only 12 years old. She was away on vacation with her parents for a few months prior to her first treatment visit. It was during this family trip that her parents noticed that she was looking very frail, and they became concerned about her increasing "fussiness" over eating and her insistence on exercising at least once every day. At the time Miranda's parents first brought her in for treatment, there were also some early signs that this prepubertal young girl was a very determined, hardworking, fastidious, and even overorganized person. In addition to being supportive and understanding toward members of the family, given the crisis they were all facing, one of the first goals of treatment was to guide the parents in helping Miranda get her weight back on track. Without this weight gain, Miranda would not have a fair chance of entering her anticipated growth spurt as she approached menarche. Moreover, without weight recovery (and continued weight gain, given that she was only 12 and needed to gain weight throughout adolescence), her body wouldn't receive the trigger that she was healthy enough to start her first period.

Although weight gain was proceeding well, it became evident that there was another difficulty at hand that might seriously complicate the family's ability to remain focused (for now) on the job of getting Miranda's physiological and psychological development back on track. Miranda was becoming increasingly ritualistic in almost all of her behaviors. What this meant in terms of her day-to-day life was that the mere act of walking to school became an ordeal, for she couldn't step on cracks in the sidewalk. At school, she could look only at some kids but not at others. At home, she had to arrange and rearrange her room several times a day to get it "just right." Most of these rituals, together with the repeated thoughts that "I must think 'good' things," kept her from any weight gain, or at least Miranda was convinced this was true.

Of course, all these activities made a routine day very hard for everyone in the family and left Miranda very little time to enjoy being with her parents and siblings, visiting with friends, or doing any homework. At this point, understanding these thoughts and rituals better so that appropriate treatment could be started had to be added to an already stressful treatment regimen of weight restoration and medical follow-up.

Several more assessments were added to everyone's busy schedule, including more visits to the pediatrician and even the neurologist. A brain scan was completed to make sure that nothing was overlooked in trying to make sense of the increasingly debilitating obsessive–compulsive symptoms. Different combinations of powerful drugs, with potentially serious side effects, were started, all in the attempt to help Miranda gain some control over the intrusive thoughts and tiring rituals. All in all, her treatment became very complicated, and Miranda, her parents, and even the treatment team had trouble managing all the different components.

Obsessive–compulsive disorder, as in Miranda's case, seems to occur commonly with eating disorders, especially anorexia, in just over one-third of patients with chronic anorexia, according to one report. Because addressing these debilitating symptoms involves a great deal of extra attention from the treatment team, such as additional interventions—cognitive-behavioral therapy and often several medications—it is easy to see how the focus could be diverted from Miranda's self-starvation. The challenge here is to address the comorbid illness but not lose track of the primary job: taking care of the eating disorder.

Depression is another psychiatric illness quite likely to occur in combination with a child's eating disorder. According to one study, as many as 63% of all patients with eating disorders have a lifetime history of depression. It's important, however, to determine whether the co-occurring depression is a primary (independent) diagnosis or the result (side effect) of self-starvation—a question best sorted out by your teen's psychiatrist or psychologist. Although it will not always be easy for your child's doctor to distinguish between these two forms of mood disturbance, effective treatment of your adolescent will depend on a careful and accurate evaluation of her mood.

Clinical depression and low mood because of an eating disorder are two different things, even though they may look very similar to you. If your child, in addition to her eating disorder, suffers from clinical depression, the depression may respond to medication, or it may persist even when the eating disorder has responded to treatment. Keep in mind, though, that many eating-disordered adolescents appear dysphoric and demoralized. This form of "depression" may certainly be the result of the eating disorder, inasmuch as poor mood is a frequent side effect of starvation. The same is true when your child engages in binge eating and purging: She could very well feel "blue," guilty, disgusted, demoralized, sad, and so forth, because of these symptoms.

For clinical depression, you should make sure your child's psychiatrist considers psychotherapy specifically for the depression, and in some instances psychotherapy plus an antidepressant, as the primary treatment. If you and your child's doctor are convinced that her low mood is secondary to her eating disorder symptoms, you should monitor her mood closely to be sure it also improves as her eating disorder is getting better. If that doesn't happen, additional treatment for the depressed mood might be in order.

Some researchers in this field argue that, in addition to obsessive–compulsive disorder and depression, there is a higher than expected comorbidity between **personality disorders** and eating disorders. For instance, avoidant personality (characterizing someone who is overcautious when it comes to interpersonal relationships, who finds it extremely difficult to make friends and is very shy, etc.) and anorexia often co-occur, and a significant number of individuals with bulimia have borderline personality (are very impulsive in their behaviors and have changeable moods as well as great instability in relationships). Although this may be the case for adults with eating disorders, it's unclear whether a finding of personality disorder *and* an eating disorder is applicable to adolescents or children. The reason we're uncertain is that doctors usually won't diagnose adolescents with a personality disorder until they reach at least 18 years of age—personality isn't something that establishes itself firmly until adulthood.

Nonetheless, many researchers from a number of theoretical backgrounds have reported differences in personality makeup among teens with various eating disorders. What many of them show is that anorexic girls are often very anxious, inhibited, and regimented, whereas bulimic adolescents can be all of these, but some also tend to be more emotionally volatile, impulsive, and/or uninhibited.

You should, however, keep two things in mind when trying to get an idea of how likely it is that your child—or any child—has other psychological problems along with an eating disorder. First, we'd be oversimplifying the eating disorders if we were to box anorexic and bulimic teens into two neat categories. Second, it is also possible that current studies overestimate comorbid illness among individuals with an eating disorder. It may be that many eating-disordered patients who are included in research projects come from specialized eating disorder clinics, and therefore the more seriously compromised individuals may be overrepresented among those studied. In reality, children and adolescents with eating disorders are quite varied, and although many of them have comorbid illnesses, many do not. For you as a parent, the important point is to be aware of the possibility and alert to signs that something else may need the attention of your child's mental health care team.

Finally, **alcohol and drug abuse** are also commonly diagnosed in adults with bulimia, though no studies have documented this in younger patients. Many teens, however, start experimenting with alcohol and drugs, and your child may not be different. If your child has both bulimia and substance use difficulties, treatment can be considerably complicated. We have mentioned that bulimia can be quite a secretive illness, which already complicates your involvement in trying to help your child. When the eating disorder coexists with another secretive problem such as drug taking, your adolescent child will be very reluctant to have you "interfere" with any of these behaviors. You will have to approach your child very carefully under these circumstances, for you might have to follow a narrow line between convincing your teen that you want to help and antagonizing your child because he or she perceives you as interfering.

Notwithstanding the sparse information about comorbid psychiatric illness among adolescents with eating disorders, if we borrow from the adult literature as well as from our own clinical experience, it seems clear that the eating disorders are indeed becoming more heterogeneous. That means there is not a "typical" eating-disordered adolescent, and these illnesses often appear along with other psychiatric illnesses. Certainly, this makes our understanding of eating disorders more complex, and, as we've demonstrated, it inevitably complicates treatment further. A final example demonstrates this point well:

> Tina had had bulimia since she was 13 and rapidly exhibited a range of other psychiatric problems. First, she became increasingly confrontational and difficult with her parents, then she began skipping school to meet boys in the park, where she smoked marijuana and drank shots. At first these activities, like her bulimia, were kept secret from her family, but over time her parents caught on. However, by that point Tina was already drinking heavily and experimenting with crack cocaine. She needed treatment in a substance abuse program before directing attention to her bulimia was even considered.

At this point there should be no doubt in your mind that eating disorders are serious illnesses that require serious attention. Think of the title of Chapter 1 as your clarion call. Go back to the warning signs and "act-now" signs listed on pages 21–22. If your child fits these descriptions, take action before an eating disorder does any more damage to your child's health. If you're concerned that your child may suffer from something other than an eating disorder, seek treatment so that these problems are prevented from doing additional harm.

It won't be easy. As you probably already know, the nature of eating disorders pits you against your child, because the eating disorder wants to stay in control. If you're to have the best possible chance of setting your child on the road to recovery quickly, you'll have to get into your child's head to get an idea of how the eating disorder is actually experienced by your son or daughter. Knowing how an eating disorder changes your teenager's thinking, attitudes, and behaviors will help you fight for your child's life.

FOR MORE INFORMATION

Mitchell, J., C. Pomeroy, and D. Adson, Managing Medical Complications, in D. M. Garner and P. E. Garfinkel, Editors, *Handbook of Treatment for Eating Disorders*, Second Edition, 1997. New York: Guilford Press, pp. 383–393.

Palmer, B., *Helping People with Eating Disorders: A Clinical Guide to Assessment and Treatment*, 2000. Chichester, England: Wiley.

Powers, P., Management of Patients with Comorbid Medical Conditions, in D. M. Garner and P. E. Garfinkel, Editors, *Handbook of Treatment for Eating Disorders*, Second Edition, 1997. New York: Guilford Press, pp. 424–436.

Zipfel, S., B. Lowe, and W. Herzog, Medical Complications, in J. Treasure, U. Schmidt, and E. van Furth, Editors, *Handbook of Eating Disorders*, 2003. Chichester, England: Wiley, pp. 169–190.

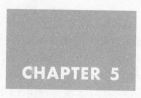

CHAPTER 5

GET INTO YOUR CHILD'S HEAD
The Distorted Thinking
Behind Your Teenager's Behavior

If your daughter or son has an eating disorder or seems to be developing one, you've probably already been told many times, "You don't understand me" or, in fact, "Nobody understands me." This feeling is very real for someone who is struggling with an eating disorder, and it's possible that you've become very frustrated trying to understand your daughter or son. Trying to communicate your position to your troubled child can be even more problematic.

The fact is that you may *not* understand what your child is experiencing. Children and adolescents with eating disorders see their behavior—especially behavior related to food, eating, weight, exercise, and health—quite differently from the way it looks from the outside. Eating disorders alter logical ways of thinking about food and body image. They distort what your son or daughter sees in the mirror. They implant in your child's mind irrational expectations about the consequences of eating and not eating, exercising and not exercising.

Unless you begin to understand how your teenager's thinking has been affected by the eating disorder, your efforts to be supportive of your child's struggle against the illness will be handicapped. You may be reading your child's behavior as non-sensical or defiant, when she sees perfect sense in it and is not trying to make you feel bad but hoping to make herself feel good. It may seem irrefutably clear to you that your child is ema-ciated and dangerously ill, but how can you hope to get her to change her behavior if you don't realize that she still sees a fat person in the mirror and feels proud of herself for sticking to her "diet"?

Your child sees herself and all things food-related through a lens imposed by the eating disorder. We call the thoughts that emerge through this lens *cognitive distortions*. In this chapter we explore the cognitive distortions that are driving your child's behavior so you can see things the way she does and thus know better how to respond constructively.

A SHIFT IN ATTITUDE, A NEW APPROACH

Before delving into specific cognitive distortions that you may be trying to deal with every day, think for a minute about the strat-egy you've been using in trying to resolve your teenager's disor-dered eating. Have you been trying to "talk some sense" into your daughter? Or are you assuming that your adolescent thinks the same way you and everyone else does when informed by common sense and reason? Now is the time to recognize that helping a child recover from an eating disorder requires, first and foremost, a new set of assumptions and a new strategy.

Understanding exactly how your child with an eating disor-der is thinking is a challenge. In fact, it is often quite tricky for doctors to fully understand just how the mind of an adolescent with anorexia or bulimia works in regard to the issues of eating, weight, and dieting. Yes, you should try to develop an under-standing of the ways of thinking that guide your child's behavior. But you won't always be able to fathom what makes her do what she does or feel how she feels. So the safest strategy for parents to take is to *assume*, as hard as this may be for you, that your ado-lescent's thinking with respect to weight and shape issues is probably almost always distorted. This is especially true with anorexia.

It will also be helpful in coping with your child's illness not to underestimate just how firmly lodged these mental distortions are. It's easy to underestimate the intransigence of these distortions, and you will often be tempted to talk some sense into your child. After all, it all seems so clear to you. Watching your child struggle to eat what appears to be a perfectly reasonable portion of food, for example, could certainly lead you to think or say, "Why not just eat it? It's so easy." Likewise, parents with an anorexic teen find themselves exhausted after lengthy, and fruitless, arguments, having tried to convince their child that a salad with dressing won't be harmful. The parents of an adolescent with bulimia may discover that their child has made herself sick in the bathroom and might very well be tempted to advise her to "just stop doing it," adding, "It'll be easy: Just get some self-control." It is, of course, not easy at all—not for you or for your child. Both anorexia and bulimia exert such a firm grip on your child's thinking that most of your pleading or arguing will be in vain.

We like to refer to such discussions as "anorexic debate" or "bulimic debate"—parents trying, in a very rational way, to convince the child that eating is good for her or that she needs the salad or that the meal the parent so painstakingly prepared won't be harmful. Most of the time, parents lose these debates. The thinking of someone with an eating disorder is so firmly lodged in cognitive distortions that there is no way you are going to argue your child out of her eating disorder. Someone with anorexia won't understand your perfectly logical argument about why this or that food item should be eaten. The beans, rice, or chicken you know will be nutritious for your child simply fills her with horror, because the food is "bad," "fattening," "unnecessary," "not the right food group," "scary," or deemed unacceptable in some other way.

When you find yourself tempted to try to reason with your child in these debates, it may help to keep one fact firmly in mind: *These cognitive distortions are usually the side effects of starvation, and dislodging such beliefs through rational debate is all but fruitless.* No doubt you were shocked by the long list of medical consequences of starvation that you read in Chapter 4. Cognitive distortions are another serious consequence, possibly the most ominous of all, because this is the one that keeps the eating disorder going. Restoring weight will certainly help in this matter, but we'll get to how that happens later on.

Teenagers with bulimia have many of the same concerns about what food may "do to them" as those with anorexia. Some subtle differences may center on "forbidden foods." This is not to say that someone with anorexia would not have a long list of "forbidden foods"—quite the opposite—it's just that for those with bulimia, there are very definite foods they believe are "forbidden" because they know eating these in particular will set off a binge that will be followed by purging. Because this chain of events is all too familiar to your child with bulimia, these particular foods are avoided at all costs!

COGNITIVE DISTORTIONS:
HOW THINGS LOOK TO YOUR CHILD
AS COMPARED WITH HOW THEY LOOK TO YOU

Accepting the fact that the eating disorder itself is making it impossible for your child to grasp reality and embrace logic in food-related matters confers a couple of important benefits:

1. It helps you separate the illness from your teenager and thereby remain as compassionate and empathetic as possible as you guide your child toward recovery. Interpreting refusal to eat, or denial of what the mirror declares, as defiance or some other willful negative behavior is counterproductive, only reinforcing the adversarial relationship on which the eating disorder thrives. We discuss this further a little later in this chapter and in Chapter 7 as well.

2. It allows you to shift your attention to exploring the specific ways in which your child thinks differently from you, which in turn will give you ideas for fighting the eating disorder in everyday situations. The rest of this chapter is devoted to the common cognitive distortions that come with eating disorders, with general suggestions for how to respond constructively. Part III of this book goes into more detail on applying this knowledge to individual situations.

It's killing her, but your daughter feels good about refusing to eat, because it's something she does well.

Adolescents who have eating disorders, especially those with anorexia nervosa, are usually quite driven in nature. You can't just get "a little" anorexia; you have to be "perfect" at having anorexia. In fact, you have to be better at having anorexia than any other adolescent with this illness. We often see girls with anorexia who, when told they need inpatient care, burst into tears in our office, saying, " But I will be the 'fattest' anorexic on the ward!" or "I can't go there—I won't be as 'good' as the others."

Adolescents with anorexia have usually been praised for their ability to be "determined," "focused," and "energetic," not for their anorexia, of course, but for their performance at math, cross-country, or just about anything they put their minds to. Many parents describe their teen with anorexia this way: "Once he's decided to do anything, there's no way you're going to deter him," or, "When he goes for something, he gives it all he has." This quality usually leads to numerous healthy achievements in school, sports, and other extracurricular activities. The difficulty arises when everyone other than your child—you, his teachers, and his peers—recognizes these achievements, but he does not. For someone with anorexia, achievements are soon forgotten, but failures (real or perceived—getting an A– as opposed to an A+) are mulled over and quickly blot out any prior accomplishments.

This all-or-nothing thinking can be devastating. Susan works very hard at being the perfect student, does her work meticulously every day, has no time to go out in the evenings or even on weekends, and has an "unblemished" report card that is a strong reminder to her that she is a "good" person and that others will like her. Without that, she'll be "nothing," "worthless," and an "utter failure." So when she was given a B in calculus the other day, her first B ever, she was devastated. She came home sobbing, telling her parents that "things will never be the same again," "no one will ever speak to me again," and she was a "miserable failure," "dumb, stupid," and "useless!"

What often happens is that a young person with anorexia really thinks she is in fact a "loser," "good at nothing," "unattractive," and so on, when she doesn't achieve just as much as she has set out to achieve. The bar is always set high and is constantly being raised, all in an effort to convince herself that she is indeed worthy. Hilde Bruch, a famous psychiatrist who wrote extensively about issues such as self-esteem in persons with anorexia (see Chapter 3), talked about this focus on one's failures as an "overwhelming sense of ineffectiveness."

As a result, and for reasons we don't fully understand, dieting may seem like an attractive solution to your child—something she thinks will "really help me feel better about myself." This may especially be the route she is attracted to when she thinks she's good at nothing else, and she thinks she's overweight, or someone at school made a derogatory comment about her weight, or so many other teens are on diets and it seems like a good thing to do. Because your child has this ability to do whatever she does well, or to go all out, she will set her mind on dieting or exercising, or both, well too. Unfortunately, when she starts succeeding at dieting and/or exercise and starts losing weight, she may be encouraged by the way she looks, by the positive reinforcement she may be getting from peers, from her family, by her improved performance at cross-country running, and so on. It seems easy then for this achievement to supplant most other achievements, and it soon becomes the only thing your child thinks she does well.

In fact, anorexia nervosa is often associated with an immense sense of pride: "I can say no to food when everyone else does not have such will power" or "I can lose weight successfully when all of you are struggling just to shed a pound" or "I can run this extra mile even though I have not eaten much all day—none of you would be able to do that." This sense of "better than you" might be subtle, but if it's the only thing your teen thinks she's good at, she will do everything to defend it. Thus, soon this ability to go without food is seen as her only sense of accomplishment, and anyone who attempts to persuade her to gain weight is seen as ignorant at best, but most likely as cruel and insensitive. It therefore feels incongruous when others criticize the teenager for being such a successful dieter (something many peers and parents have failed at) or try to "derail" his twice-daily routine of 200 crunches, 200 push-ups, 200 sit-ups, and so on. Your child feels that others simply envy him or her.

Again, the struggle for most parents is tackling this relent-lessness that is so characteristic of eating disorders, without feel-ing as if they are taking something perceived to be so precious away from their child. Indeed, most teens with anorexia nervosa will make parents feel as if they're being most unkind in getting them to gain weight, while the parents will have to find a way to persevere in their efforts to help their child redirect her ability to be a "good anorexic" into another, much more fruitful and healthier endeavor.

Your child's behavior demonstrates that she's out of control, but she sees it as a way to stay in charge and express her independence.

In the usual pursuit of autonomy, there are many ways in which adolescents seek control of their own lives: choosing their own friends, driving themselves where they need to go, setting their own standards of performance, and so on. However, when ado-lescents' choices indicate they are not in control—binge drinking, serious risk-taking behavior, *and* anorexia and bulimia nervosa, to name just a few examples—the issue for parents is clearly how to set appropriate limits on independence and control. When dieting leads to anorexia, the adolescent needs help to reestab-lish normal adolescent autonomy processes and experimenta-tion, and the options available do not include food restriction. The same is true when food restriction leads to bouts of binge eating, followed by purging, as is the case with bulimia: Parents often have to assist the adolescent in normalizing eating (three healthy meals per day) so that other aspects of adolescent experi-mentation do not also suffer as a consequence of the lack of con-trol over eating.

The challenge for most of you, though, is that although the child's behavior demonstrates that she is out of control, your son or daughter will more than likely see the eating disorder as the only way to stay in charge and express some independence.

Your teenager will vigorously fend off any attempts you might make to help. There will be little you can do that won't be perceived as "you're always telling me what to do" or "you always want to control my every move."

Anorexia may look somewhat different from bulimia here. Adolescents with anorexia will probably come across as quite "together" or "in control" of their lives. In fact, the illness is often associated with a great sense of order, neatness, and discipline. Grades in school continue to be high. All of this serves to confuse most parents as they contemplate the fact that their child is perhaps not in charge of things. We've often heard parents say, "Yes, she's 17 and weighs 82 pounds, but her grades are excellent, she's really working hard, and she's doing so well." The dilemma is made even more difficult by the fact that your daughter with anorexia will assert, repeatedly, that she is fine, that she is in control, and that she can make her own decisions in a rational way. Your daughter will even be so persuasive in her arguments that you will find it hard not to believe her. The irony is that the illness also has the ability to convince the adolescent that she is indeed in charge of her eating and weight management and that she can stop dieting and lose weight anytime she wants—"just not now!"

"I can take care of this myself" is also very persuasive to most parents, frightened about what they think might happen to their child but desperate in their willingness to believe that she can get better by herself, as she's repeatedly assured them she can. However, the way the physiology and psychology of starvation work is that at a certain point, usually once weight loss has clearly begun, the adolescent loses control over this process and cannot stop dieting, or get herself to eat a decent amount of food, even if she *wants* to. The anorexia has firmly established its own control over the thinking and behavior of your adolescent.

This is a critical point to remember at all times: *Once your child has reached the point of significant weight loss, she usually cannot get better by herself, even if she proclaims that she can.* As a parent, it's important for you to realize that this doesn't necessarily mean she does not want to get better. It's just that the anorexia is more powerful as an illness than your child's solo efforts at defeating the illness. Remember your new set of assumptions when you're tempted to fall back into the attitude that your child is just being obstinate and all it will take for her to start eating normally again is for you to talk some sense into her.

Again, the only way to get your child out of this dilemma is for you and her treatment team to help her restore her weight. *It is only with weight restoration that she will think in healthy and rational ways, and it is only with weight restoration that she will have a chance to get back on track with adolescent development and achieve healthy and appropriate control over her individuation and budding independence.*

Bulimia is not altogether different, but with this illness it may be easier for you to notice that your adolescent is indeed out of control. You can probably think of many times that you've missed a box of cookies from the pantry: You knew it was there just this morning, and now it's gone. You remember putting last night's leftover chicken in the fridge, and now it's missing. You've noticed the candy wrappers in the trash in Maggie's room every day! And you've also spotted the remnants of her purging in the bathroom, week after week now.

Many adolescents with bulimia may feel ambivalent about anyone interfering with their attempts to control their weight, their eating, and even their purging, but are in fact quite relieved when a parent helps them succeed in breaking the shameful pattern of binge eating and purging. Another difference in bulimia. as compared with anorexia, is that your teenager with bulimia will not so stridently insist that she is in control of her eating. In fact, every time she has a binge-eating episode followed by purging, whether it is self-induced vomiting or laxative or diuretic abuse, your daughter feels more and more out of control: "I feel disgusted with myself every time I do this, but I just don't know how to stop. I am so afraid that I will gain weight if I don't make myself sick, and that's why I just can't stop doing this." However, many other teens are more likely to deny feeling out of control, especially as they'll probably make every effort to reestablish control over eating *after* a binge/purge episode. Unlike that of a teen with anorexia, this sense of control seldom lasts for more than a couple of days, only to be followed by binge eating and purging again. Nevertheless, your daughter with bulimia is probably more likely to assert that she is, in fact, in control of her behavior and that it isn't up to you to tell her what to do about her difficulties. This is particularly confusing to you as a parent, as you've seen your child acting quite independently in so many other areas of her adolescence. Helping her with her bulimia now seems almost counterintuitive!

Whether your child has anorexia or bulimia, it is highly likely that he won't think he is out of control and will probably resent you for trying to help. The challenge for you is how you will delicately balance your understanding of your teenager's developmental needs for independence with your understanding of his dilemma and find a way to help him assert healthy control over his life at a time he might resent you for your "interference." What is clear, though, is that you don't really have a choice. You have to help your child as the eating disorder continues to cloud his judgment.

To you, this is a deadly disease; to your child, it's "just a perfectly healthy diet."

You now realize just how devastating an eating disorder is, but to see your child being flippant about her low heart rate, anemia, blood in her vomit, and swollen parotid glands is to come face-to-face with one of the most alarming aspects of anorexia and bulimia—the inability of the person with the eating disorder to appreciate just how deadly these illnesses can be. This denial of the seriousness of the severe malnutrition associated with anorexia nervosa is a core symptom of the illness. Teens with bulimia nervosa will not necessarily understand the seriousness of their symptoms either, especially purging behaviors and their potentially serious health consequences. Someone with anorexia does not appreciate how lethal severe emaciation can be, and similarly, someone with bulimia does not understand that low potassium, due to frequent vomiting for instance, can cause his or her death. It's fair to say, though, that this denial is perhaps a little more pronounced in anorexia.

In Chapter 4 we explained that anorexia is an ego-syntonic illness. What this means is that, unlike those with many other mental disorders, the patient with anorexia "likes" or "cherishes" the illness or "takes comfort" in the illness. Someone with anorexia doesn't appreciate its dangers and will do almost any-thing to protect it, that is, prevent you from "taking it away." Although parents and doctors alike find this aspect of anorexia very difficult to understand, it helps to think of anorexia in comparison with other mental disorders: The patient who is depressed wants to feel better, the person who is anxious wants to relax, but the person with anorexia still wants to be thinner. This denial is actually reinforced through constant dieting and further weight loss, as well as focusing on these issues (dieting and weight) all the time to the exclusion of other, healthier per-spectives. Thus, her diet is still normal to your daughter, even though everyone else sees it for what it is. Therefore, it's not uncommon for someone with anorexia to take pride in brushes with death: "Wow, I got my potassium down to 1.8, and I made it" (showing up in the emergency room with a potassium level that low is considered most critical, and few people can be revived).

What makes this illness so incredibly dangerous is that no matter how much you argue this very point with your teenager with anorexia—"You could have died . . . We are so lucky they managed to revive you at the hospital . . . We were so, so scared . . . Do you understand how serious this is?"—these facts usually will have little impact on your son or daughter. Quietly, he or she'll perceive this "crisis" as another achievement in his or her quest for that ideal weight.

By comparison, bulimia is ego-dystonic. What this means is that although an adolescent with bulimia exhibits many of the aspects of denial of her illness that are common in anorexia, there is less pride involved in her symptoms. Rather, great dis-comfort and shame are associated with binge eating and purg-ing. Nevertheless, this doesn't mean that your son or daughter will be forthcoming and ask for help as an adolescent who is depressed or anxious might. Quite the opposite is true. Because thinness is highly valued and the seriousness of the illness is not appreciated, *and* because of the guilt and shame associated with bulimic symptoms, most adolescents will do their best to binge eat without your knowledge and purge while "taking a shower." Their anxiety that the food they ate will make them gain 5 pounds overnight is so overwhelming that they absolutely "have to" get rid of it and will make every effort to make sure there's a way to purge after the binge-eating episodes. It certainly is not uncommon for a teenager to evaluate an invitation for a movie and a meal with his or her friends, based not on what movie they'll see or what kind of food (Asian, Italian, etc.) they'll eat, but rather on the answers to questions like, "Will I be able to purge at that restaurant?" or "Can I slip away at that movie house to use the bathroom to throw up?"

As has probably become clear by now, gaining a better understanding of how the eating disorder leads your child to think and behave in very fixed ways concerning weight, shape, and eating issues will be helpful to you in finding the right way to help your adolescent overcome this struggle. That doesn't mean this understanding will automatically suggest an instantly effective strategy; it's just that without this understanding you're unlikely even to know why your efforts fail. Chapters 7 and 8 offer various ideas for helping your child, based on your understanding of these cognitive distortions.

You're the enemy, even though you're trying to save your son's life, because you're "forcing" him to do the one thing he is trying to avoid: eat.

The cognitive distortions born of eating disorders, by their very nature, create an adversarial relationship between you and your child. You want the child to eat appropriately to regain his health; he is firmly committed to continuing to lose weight or to hide the truth that he is binge eating and purging. The fact that you can't "talk some sense into him" means that any attempt on your part to confront your child's false beliefs and consequent denial only make you seem like a greater enemy.

The rift between you may seem to widen from your own perspective too when you try to confront your teenager about irrational beliefs surrounding food and weight. You may very well have come to count on the rational discussion and sharing of decision making that are among the beneficial developments of life with an adolescent. In fact, you may feel today that you have a perfectly rational adolescent around the house most of the time—"We can talk about homework, our vacation plans, or the music she likes to listen to"—but when it comes to food and weight issues, "it's as if a switch was turned off: She makes no sense, and the worst is, she doesn't see the difference." The fact that your teenager is no longer meeting your expectations for rationality may make you feel as if it's the child who is creating the adversarial situation. With this kind of standoff, who wins?

The eating disorder wins.

That's because the real—and only—enemy is the anorexia or the bulimia. Recognizing this is the key to responding constructively to this particular cognitive distortion.

The thought distortions associated with eating disorders can be so severe that rational discussion and decision sharing about your child's health are no longer possible. Parents have to be prepared to accept the idea that in the area of food, eating, and weight, they are no longer dealing with a child who is rational. It is the *illness* they are dealing with.

We've seen many parents in distress when their usually kind adolescent lashes out when his parents make any attempt to intervene in the illness: "I don't want to eat that! You're killing me. Can't you see how unhappy you make me?" or "I hate you, I want nothing to do with you, don't even talk to me!" or "Leave me alone! You are making me *soo* miserable." Desperate utterances from your adolescent sounding anything like these are obviously distressing to any parent. What the adolescent with anorexia or bulimia wants is for you to back off in your efforts to help. As tempting as this might be for many parents, acquiescing only means allowing the illness to triumph.

What can you do? Negotiating with your adolescent under these circumstances is a great challenge and one that you are most likely to lose. In defense of his illness, your son will try to make sure that your efforts fail, whether you are trying to get him to eat more or to keep him from purging the food that he has consumed. Knowing that there is little you can do to rationally argue, discuss, or convince your son about the perils of his illness and that the behaviors he is manifesting are illness related as opposed to those of "your child" (separating the illness from your adolescent) will help you when you're trying to help him. Knowing that getting involved in "eating disorder debates" will be fruitless and that you will probably lose the argument and end up being convinced, against your own better judgment, that an apple is better than a pasta dish with a cream sauce for a starving teenager, it's best not to argue. Instead, you will want to find a way to let your child know that you understand his dilemma, that the illness doesn't allow him to be rational about food and weight right now, that you understand that for the time being he sees you as the enemy, but that none of this can deter you from doing what you know will save his life—to get him to eat what he should eat, or to keep him from binge eating and purging.

Earlier we mentioned the concept of separating the illness from your adolescent. This is an important principle in dealing with a teenager with an eating disorder, just as it is in helping someone of any age with any psychiatric disorder. Understanding how the illness is "separate" from your teenager will be crucial in helping you understand your child's troubled behaviors and deal with the illness effectively. We discuss this principle in more detail in Chapter 7.

"Not eating" is not just the most important thing in your daughter's life; it's "the only thing."

For parents, it is often very difficult to understand just how important eating or not eating, weight loss, or feeling the "right" size is to their daughter. In fact, for someone with anorexia, nothing can be more important than focusing on that next pound that she should lose or making sure that she doesn't eat at all until 5:00 P.M. every day of the next week. For someone with bulimia, nothing can be more important than how he or she can get rid of the food he or she has just eaten, believing it's going to make him or her fat. Indeed, managing to adhere to all these "rules" and "regulations" around eating or not eating eventually eclipses the importance of school, family, and friends, or at least it appears to do so, especially if the eating disorder behaviors are allowed to continue unchecked. It is especially hard for parents to witness their kind child appear completely oblivious to other crises in the family—it's not uncommon for an adolescent with anorexia to show little concern for a parent who was just diag-

nosed with a severe illness, because the adolescent is so preoccupied with his or her quest for thinness. This adolescent is,
of course, not heartless; it's just that anorexia or bulimia has a
way of overtaking the sufferer, leaving little room for anything
else.

Paradoxically, when someone with anorexia continues to
starve himself, it actually becomes easier and easier not to eat. At
the onset of the illness the adolescent has to work very hard to
keep her appetite "in check," making sure she doesn't "give in"
to these "horrible urges" to eat, always feeling that she cannot let
her guard down for a moment. With increasing weight loss,
though, it becomes easier to feel a sense of mastery over these
urges, and with time the teenager no longer feels any hunger.
However, with increased starvation, the adolescent also becomes
more preoccupied with thoughts about food and weight. In fact,
some young women and men find themselves in the unenviable
position where they can think of virtually nothing else but "What
is that half bagel from this morning going to do to my weight?"
or "What can I do to avoid having lunch with my friends?" or
"How can I make sure that I have no more than a salad without
dressing for dinner?" and so on. It's hard to imagine just how
much of one's time, on a daily basis, will be taken up by such
thoughts. Some teens with anorexia will say, "I can think of nothing else but my weight, literally nothing else!"

Much of what happens with the dieting adolescent, especially when starvation has set in, also happens to people who lose
extreme amounts of weight because of a variety of medical illnesses. In fact, much of what we know about the effects of starvation on the human mind and on human behavior is derived from
what we have learned from individuals without an eating disorder. Ancel Keys and his colleagues, in a landmark study in
Minnesota in the early 1950s, published their results of a
semistarvation study of World War II conscientious objectors.
The physical and psychological changes in these healthy men
who were starved for several months were the same as those we
typically observe in our patients with an eating disorder—the
men became increasingly preoccupied with their weight and
with food once they had lost a substantial amount of weight. It's
almost as if the part of the brain that controls hunger and satiety

will not let you forget about the one thing you need most when you're starved—food! The good news is that once these starved study participants were allowed to eat normally again, their weights were restored and the symptoms of starvation also disappeared. These observations reveal exactly what we also witness in many patients with anorexia when they return to a healthy weight.

Your daughter has consumed mere crumbs of food, but she thinks she's telling the truth when she says she's eaten a huge amount of food today.

When your adolescent has consumed only a few bites of her sandwich and proclaims to have eaten "tons" or "too much" or a "huge amount," there are at least two ways in which her account is accurate from her perspective. First, she sees eating anything at all as a failure and a sign of weakness. So, psychologically, even a small amount is the same as a large amount to her. The anxiety and guilt she experiences after eating half a bagel are the same as if she had eaten a whole sandwich. Second, and in reality, the stomach of someone with anorexia usually decreases in capacity, and as a consequence, the rate at which the stomach empties has been slowed. It's therefore quite likely that your child will feel full and stay feeling that way longer after eating even a relatively small amount of food. Moreover, prolonged starvation has allowed your teenager's hunger cues to have been stilled, making eating even more difficult when she states that she's not hungry. So, when she does eat, even what are in fact mere crumbs, your daughter will feel that she has overeaten on both accounts. "I will get fat if I eat that bagel (half an apple/ three carrots/etc.)", she will say, or "I just can't eat that much, I've already had enough," in reference to the small bowl of salad without dressing that sits half eaten. These incidents are, in fact, experienced by your child as really having eaten too much or really finding it hard to eat the "whole" salad.

The situation is further complicated when parents want to believe their adolescent's account of what was eaten when they (the parents) weren't around to supervise a meal. And parents can become increasingly despondent when their child doesn't gain weight despite "all the food" she claims to be eating on a regular basis. It is very important for you to remember that eating even half an apple at school lunch, when your adolescent son has promised himself not to eat at all, is seen by him as a calamitous transgression of his own food rules and that the half apple was a huge amount of food—"huge" because it "should not have been eaten." Likewise, asking your adolescent daughter to tell you what she ate for lunch at school might get you a response along these lines: "A yogurt and chips and a milkshake." That may sound like enough, but if you inquire carefully, it may in fact mean that in reality, she ate a scoop of yogurt, a bite of an apple, and a sip of a milkshake. As has become clear to you by now, even when your child protests about "too much food" or says, "I can't possible have more to eat," recovery from anorexia can really come about only when sufficiently healthy amounts of food are consumed to return your child's thinking about these issues to normal and, of course, to restore gut functioning to normal.

The same scenario may be true for an adolescent with bulimia, but it will take a slightly different form. Whereas your teen with bulimia will also try to restrict her food intake and may also consider mere crumbs of food "a lot," many teens with bulimia are very scared that if they eat "one more crumb" than their self-imposed food rules allow, they will "just go ahead and eat the whole cake." Sadly, that is what happens for many teens with bulimia, and that's why your child will so rigidly try to hang on to these beliefs.

No matter how emaciated she becomes, what your daughter sees in the mirror is a fat person.

This is called *body image distortion*, which is a result of an overfocus on weight and shape that eventually leads to misapprehension of realities. Many teenagers with anorexia overestimate their own body size, and quite paradoxically, the thinner they become, the more they may see themselves as fat. Body image distortion is much less common among those with bulimia. Some teenagers may go so far as to cover all mirrors in their homes so they can never catch a glimpse of themselves. There are sophisticated methods whereby body image distortion can be evaluated. However, you only need to hear your child referring to herself as fat, or have her tell you what she sees when she looks in the mirror, to know that she actually sees someone who is much larger than she actually is.

Unfortunately, the only "solution" your son or daughter can think of to escape this agonizing dilemma is to lose yet another pound, thereby establishing a cycle of further weight loss and further distortion of reality. One insightful teenage patient described her experience like this: "I thought I was fat when I wore these pants. Now that I have gained weight I can't see any difference (I still look as fat), but the pants are the same. I guess I can't see things the way they really are. My fear of being fat makes me look fat no matter what."

Many teenagers, though, know they are thin and don't actually see themselves as fat, yet they still cannot escape "feeling fat." Someone might say: "I know I'm not fat, but every morning I wake up feeling fat, and I know there's only one way to tackle my problem and that's to lose more weight. Perhaps then I won't feel fat." What may be happening here for some teenagers who are predisposed to developing an eating disorder is that it's "easier" to wake up in the morning and focus on your weight than to think about "that issue at school" or "the breakup with my boyfriend." Many teenagers with eating disorders may not know how to tackle or resolve the issues that cause them to feel depressed, but it's a little "easier" to go on a diet and lose weight. So, instead of waking up saying "I am depressed" and then having to figure out how to deal with that feeling, it seems somewhat more manageable to "replace" the depression with "I feel fat," because at least "I have a plan to cut back on my food intake some more and lose another pound. Maybe then I'll feel OK." Obviously, losing that extra pound does not help with the feeling of fatness. But even with that evidence before her—that losing an extra pound doesn't eliminate her feeling of being fat—you will find it very difficult, if not impossible, to convince your daughter that she isn't fat. As long as that "feeling" persists, she will stay on the cycle of trying to lose weight and not eating will continue to cause the body image distortion that tells her loud and clear that she is fat.

Ironically, body image distortion usually, but not always, improves or even normalizes when weight is restored. (Not surprisingly, those whose thoughts about eating and weight are still distorted even after their weight is normalized usually have a poorer prognosis than those whose thought processes improve along with their weight.)

Your son continues to vomit even though his weight is clearly increasing.

One of the ironies of bulimia is that the weight-control strategy of purging is quite ineffective. It is impossible to vomit up the full amount one has eaten during an hour-long binge-eating episode—too much food has already entered the intestinal tract. Thus, a hefty percentage of these high-calorie foods remains in the system and adds weight. Over time, then, instead of losing weight, patients with bulimia tend to gain weight. However, this only adds to the urgency of their efforts to control their weight, which leads to increasing self-starvation, binge eating, and then purging. Still, they keep on doing it. Why?

The answer is, in part, that over time binge eating and purging are experienced as a coping strategy for other of life's problems. Over time, adolescents report feeling tremendous relief after purging. This reinforces the purging behaviors whether they lead to weight loss or not. Many adolescents who have been ill for a while readily admit that they know the purging does little to help them with weight control: "It's just that I have to do it. I feel much better afterward, even if that feeling doesn't last very long." So, when your son feels he didn't perform well at a wrestling meet, he may binge eat and purge. The same is true when your daughter breaks up with her boyfriend or is having academic trouble. In other words, binge eating and purging are no longer efforts at weight control alone; they are used more generally in an effort to cope with other problems of adolescence. When a behavior like binge eating and purging is being used to manage any number of types of problems, it's harder to let go of, and the "logic" that it doesn't control weight doesn't pertain.

**Your daughter seems prideful about her self-starvation,
but miserable at the same time.**

One of the hardest things to appreciate about severe dieting is
that although your son or daughter appears to be reveling in the
accomplishment of lower and lower weights, he or she is also
quite miserable. Anorexia nervosa is a really tough taskmaster.
Whenever your child eats even a small amount, she experiences
severe harassing and critical thoughts about failure and worth-
lessness. These thoughts are unrelenting and merciless. In addition, the preoccupation with eating, obsessive and repetitive
thinking about how much was eaten, how many calories, how
much weight gain, and so forth, disrupts usual thinking, making
it sometimes difficult to focus in school or during social gather-
ings. The point is, however determined and steadfast your child
appears, she is really suffering, physically and psychologically, as
a result of the punitive thinking experienced.

Adolescents with bulimia are usually filled with shame and
feelings of failure because they "give in" to eating and "purge"
even though it's disgusting. These adolescents experience a combination of guilt, shame, recrimination, and anxiety about gaining weight. It helps to have a sympathetic view of this experience, because as a parent, when your child is suffering, you want
to relieve that suffering, even if the illness behaviors are themselves frustrating and provoke anger in you.

**Your son weighs himself 10 times a day and is constantly
pinching himself to see if he has any fat despite his obvious
severe weight loss.**

Body checking and repeated weighing appear irrational to us
because we know that weights do not vary much during a day
and that pinching or repeatedly checking our appearance in the
mirror will not provide new information. However, the anxiety
about weight gain and a concomitant hyperfocus on body fat are
pervasive in adolescents with anorexia or bulimia. To combat
perceived weight gain or imagined weight gain, those with an
eating disorder look for reassurance in these constant "checking" activities, whether it's pinching the stomach or thighs a hun-

dred times a day or standing in front of the mirror for what seems like hours at a time, checking and rechecking to see whether any weight was put on. Unfortunately, the reassurance is only momentary (if at all), and they quickly need to check again. If you remember that these behaviors also reinforce the hyperfocus on shape and weight concerns, you will see why it's often necessary to find ways to help your child reduce his or her dependency on such strategies so as to reduce the child's anxiety about weight and shape. For instance, you might make this struggle a great deal easier for your child if you remove your bathroom scale. You can reassure your child that he or she will be weighed at regular intervals at the doctor's office, and it is at the doctor's office that these concerns can be addressed.

WHAT'S A PARENT SUPPOSED TO DO?

When you understand your child's thinking in regard to these issues, you've laid the foundation for whatever practical interventions you will implement to help fight your child's eating disorder. By separating the illness from your child (also called *externalizing the illness*), you support your child as a developing adolescent while insisting that she fight the eating disorder.

As we've shown, eating disorders are clearly very complicated illnesses, both in terms of the effects of starvation on the mind and the body and in terms of how coexisting psychiatric illnesses further complicate the picture. In addition, as we've seen in this chapter, how they are experienced by your child makes her thinking and behaviors appear irrational and confusing, though there is a kind of logic to them when you understand them better.

Treatment for eating disorders must respond to these complicated thoughts, behaviors, and, at times, medical problems. What this usually means is that good treatment pays attention to all aspects of these illnesses—psychological, psychiatric, medical, and nutritional. Good treatment also means that you, the parent, play an active role in helping your daughter or son receive care and that you actively participate in this care. Your involvement in treatment is particularly helpful here, as these cognitive distortions are so persistent and so powerful that someone has to be on hand to help counteract them, and, obviously, the parents (and the rest of the family) are usually the only ones routinely in the position to do this.

In the following chapter, we outline what research to date has been able to tell us about the effectiveness of the best-studied treatments for eating disorders. If you choose to have family therapy along the lines of the Maudsley approach (see Chapter 7), it will help you to use everything you now know about how your child thinks to enhance your success in taking charge of the problematic eating behavior. If you choose among other types of treatment, you can still use what you know about cognitive distortions to support the treatment team's efforts, as described in Chapter 8.

FOR MORE INFORMATION

Garner, D. M., Psychoeducational Principles in Treatment, in D. M. Garner and P. E. Garfinkel, Editors, *Handbook of Treatment for Eating Disorders*, Second Edition, 1997. New York: Guilford Press, p. 145–177.

Treasure, J., and B. Bauer, *Assessment and Motivation*, in J. Treasure, U. Schmidt, and E. van Furth, Editors, *Handbook of Eating Disorders*, 2003. Chichester, England: Wiley, pp. 219–232.

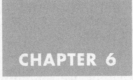

CHAPTER 6

UNDERSTAND YOUR OPTIONS

What the Research Says about the Best Ways
to Treat Anorexia and Bulimia

Having a better understanding of your adolescent's difficulties involving self-esteem, body weight, shape, and eating habits enables you to take the next step: finding help. Identifying the most appropriate treatment for your child can be a challenge, however, because researchers and the clinical community still struggle with many unknowns. Fortunately, we know more today than ever before about treatments that reverse self-starvation or binge eating and purging, that assist you and your adolescent in understanding some of the psychological makeup of his or her difficulties, and that can help get your daughter or son back on track with adolescent development.

In this chapter we present what we know about the different treatments for eating disorders. Before we get into the specifics, however, it's important to understand that the treatment studies providing evidence for the effectiveness of these therapies have mostly focused exclusively on people who meet the full criteria for either anorexia or bulimia. This does not mean that no treatment is available if your child meets the criteria for eating disorder not otherwise specified (EDNOS). Clinical experience has shown that in most settings a child whose symptoms resemble anorexia or bulimia should be treated the same way teenagers who meet the full criteria for these disorders are treated. And in some ways, the outcome might be more favorable for your child if she has been ill for only a few months or a year and does not qualify for the full diagnosis of anorexia or bulimia. *An important point to remember as you read about the available treatment options is that early and good treatment usually bodes well for your child's recovery from an eating disorder.* We start by discussing studies that evaluate outpatient approaches, then turn to more intensive therapies like inpatient, day-hospital, or residential treatments.

OUTPATIENT TREATMENTS

In this section we explain what the latest research has shown about effectiveness of the main psychological treatments for eating disorders (family therapy, psychodynamic individual therapy, cognitive-behavioral therapy, interpersonal psychotherapy, and nutritional counseling) and medication treatments.

Psychological Treatments

Because of the obvious emotional distress and needs of almost all eating disorder patients, psychological treatment is an essential component of most treatments for these problems. Yet only five controlled psychotherapy trials for adolescent eating disorders have been published as of the time of this writing. (A controlled trial is a scientifically systematic study in which patients are randomly assigned to one of at least two treatments, the treatments are quite specific, time is limited, the delivery is strictly supervised, and the outcomes are systematically compared.) Each of these studies had few participants, and all were focused on anorexia rather than bulimia. Although anorexia was first recognized at least 130 years ago and bulimia almost 25 years ago, all of these studies were conducted within the last 2 decades. Unfortunately, the studies have also produced findings that are sometimes difficult to interpret. The result is that much more research should be done to inform us all about the best treatments for these problems. It also means you should be cautious when told that someone is certain about what "the best" treatment for your child is.

Family Treatment

Because eating disorders often occur in adolescents, working with the family was identified as a possible avenue of treatment. Family therapy generally emphasizes the family system as a potential solution for the dilemmas of the eating disorder in a teenager. Although there are some important differences between early attempts to involve parents in the treatment of adolescents with eating disorders and more recent work, the groundwork was laid to bring parents very directly into the treatment process because parents are seen as most helpful in resolving the eating disorder in their adolescent. Therefore, family therapy for eating disorders has been seen as a valuable treatment since the middle 1970s.

In general family therapy, the therapist focuses on how family members communicate, how they relate to one another, and how they solve problems. The notion is that in families in which there is a member with an eating disorder, there are certain predictable problem areas such as parents allowing a child to function as an authority figure in the family, the avoidance of addressing problems in the interest of keeping the peace, and anxiety about allowing an adolescent child to be independent. The focus of this form of family therapy is not on symptoms or symptom management as in the Maudsley approach, but instead on these more general family process concerns.

Several noncontrolled trials (in which a series of patients receive the same treatment without any comparison treatment) of family therapy suggest that involving families in treatment is effective at least for younger patients with anorexia nervosa. Child psychiatrist Salvador Minuchin, who spent most of his professional life at the Child Guidance Clinic in Philadelphia, conducted the most important of these studies. He and his team reported good outcomes (recovery) in more than 85% of their patients in a case series of 53 adolescents with anorexia. All these patients were treated with family therapy. In another series of cases involving anorexia, Stierlin and Weber reported that approximately two-thirds of their patients recovered in terms of weight gain and menstruation at the time of follow-up.

The most influential systematic research into psychological treatments for eating disorders so far, however, has been the family-based treatment studies conducted at the Maudsley Hospital in London that focused on anorexia. We introduced the Maudsley approach in Chapter 2. Comparable work to that of the Maudsley doctors has been conducted, or is currently under way, in various centers in the United States. Most of these studies, in both the United Kingdom and the United States, have shown that family-based treatment can be very effective for adolescents with anorexia, especially for those who have been ill for less than 2 years. A main difference for you to remember here is that the Maudsley approach to family-based treatment, unlike many other family therapies for eating disorders, does not assume that there is something "wrong" with families or that this "something wrong" with you or your family is the reason that you should be involved in your child's treatment. On the contrary, this form of family-based treatment sees families as the best resource in treatment. Recovery of the teenager can be accelerated by successfully getting the family on board in treatment, helping the therapist to resolve the eating disorder symptoms (the starvation), and getting the adolescent back on track with adolescent development..

A randomized clinical trial from the Maudsley group compared individual therapy with family therapy. In that study, 21 teenage girls with anorexia were treated with either family therapy or supportive individual therapy. At the end of 1 year of outpatient treatment, 90% of the adolescents who received family treatment had a good outcome, as compared with only 18% of those assigned to individual therapy. In addition, in long-term follow-up, those who did well in family treatment maintained that improvement after 5 years. No other treatment for anorexia has demonstrated this level of effectiveness over the long term. The other controlled trials that have used family treatment based on the Maudsley model have found that 60–85% do well.

Although anorexia and bulimia are distinct illnesses, many adolescents with either type of eating disorder look quite alike. Therefore, in the absence of any treatment studies for adolescents with bulimia, it makes sense that family-based treatment proven effective for teenagers with anorexia may also be beneficial to your adolescent with bulimia. In addition, some case reports have been quite enthusiastic about involving families in the treatment of bulimia for adolescents and adults. As is the case with anorexia, the only evidence we have that family-based treatment may be effective in adolescents with bulimia comes from preliminary reports on treatments that have used the Maudsley approach. These investigations are encouraging. This treatment includes education about the secretiveness and seriousness of bulimia and involves parents in helping to stop their adolescent's binge/purge cycles. In most reports, young patients with bulimia responded positively and showed significant changes in bulimic symptoms from the start to the end of treatment. Further support for the use of a family approach with bulimia is derived from the studies of binge/purge-type anorexia. Two of those studies suggest that families were able to assist their children with these problems in addition to the problem of severe starvation. Although you should view these results with some caution, family treatment for adolescent bulimia has considerable potential and should be considered among your treatment options.

Individual Psychodynamic Psychotherapy

As mentioned in Chapter 2, a variety of individual psychotherapies are available, but the kind of therapy your child is most likely to receive at this time is psychodynamic therapy. This means the treatment will focus more on "underlying issues" than on weight and shape concerns and how to restore healthy body weight. This form of treatment addresses the perceived psychological problems that may cause eating disorders. Specifically, adolescents with eating disorders are believed to be immature and highly anxious about a variety of adolescent issues, including taking up independent roles as adults in a responsible manner. Therapy using this model focuses on the symptoms of disordered eating only insofar as they represent an ineffective and dangerous strategy that keeps the adolescent from addressing her real concerns and issues. Psychodynamic therapy for eating disorders is often relatively unstructured in nature, not time limited, with treatment goals that are not necessarily very specific. Nevertheless, there is some evidence to support this treatment. In two trials, Arthur Crisp and his colleagues at St. George's Hospital in London reported substantial improvements in their patient groups (these included both adolescents and adults) in terms of both medical/nutritional recovery and psychological improvement, using individual therapy approaches. Many colleagues who practice this approach are mindful of the fact that it may be difficult to do intensive psychotherapy early in treatment when someone is very starved and, consequently, will adapt their treatments to reflect this reality.

An exception to these general comments about the nonspecificity of individual psychodynamic therapy is the approach developed by Arthur Robin and colleagues at Wayne State University in Detroit, called ego-oriented individual therapy (EOIT) for anorexia. Derived from the psychodynamic tradition, EOIT aims at maturational issues associated with puberty and adolescence. EOIT devised for adolescents posits that individuals with anorexia are immature and unaware of their emotions, particularly strong emotions like anger and depression. These adolescents do not want to face such problems, so they turn to controlling food and weight as way to keep their feelings and conflicts from surfacing. Thus, according to these theories, eating disorders disrupt normal psychological and physical maturity during adolescence. To develop better ability to manage the challenges of adolescence they must first learn to identify, define, and tolerate their emotions. In addition, a primary goal of EOIT is to foster the adolescent's separation and individuation from the family.

Robin and colleagues used EIOT in a randomized clinical trial comparing it with family therapy. The comparison revealed that at the end of treatment, family therapy resulted in greater improvements, but at 1-year follow-up there were no significant differences in how patients did between the two approaches. About two-thirds of the adolescents did better overall. This study suggests that EOIT is effective, though slower in achieving results than family therapy. What may distinguish EOIT from other psychodynamic therapies is the degree to which parents are involved in the treatment, though they specifically did not directly manage eating or other compensatory behaviors like binge eating or purging.

As we noted, there are no published randomized clinical trials for adolescents with bulimia. However, there are many studies of individual therapy approaches for adults with bulimia that may be relevant to adolescents as well. The two psychological treatments in particular that have received the attention of investigators are cognitive-behavioral therapy (CBT) and interpersonal psychotherapy (IPT).

The cognitive-behavioral model of bulimia, initially developed by psychiatrist Christopher Fairburn at Oxford in England, assumes that the main factors involved in the maintenance of bulimia are problematic *attitudes* toward body shape and weight. Such attitudes lead to an overvaluation of thinness, to dissatisfaction with the body, and to attempts to control shape and weight through excessive dieting. This restrictive pattern of eating then results in both psychological and physiological deprivation, which are often associated with a depressed mood. As a result of the dietary restriction, hunger is increased, leading to an enhanced probability of binge eating, particularly in the presence of depressed mood. Because binge eating raises concerns about gaining weight, it is eventually followed by purging in an attempt to compensate for calories consumed during the binge. Using this model, treatment for bulimia using CBT focuses first on helping to change patterns of eating to make them more normal (i.e., three meals and snacks without long periods of fasting between them) so that the urge to binge eat (and therefore purge as well) is decreased. Next, the treatment focuses on the effect of overvaluation of shape and weight on self-esteem and other related thoughts that support an excessive preoccupation with these matters and lead to disordered eating behaviors. Finally, the treatment focuses on what might be expected to lead to a return of problems with eating in the future and helps to determine what might be done to prevent a relapse.

Different groups of investigators in several countries have completed a number of randomized controlled trials of CBT for bulimia. Almost all of these studies have demonstrated that CBT is the treatment of choice for adults with bulimia. More specifically, these studies have shown that CBT produces a mean reduction in binge eating and purging of about 70% and a mean abstinence rate from these symptoms approaching 50%. Dietary restraint is also lessened significantly, and the disturbed attitudes toward body weight and shape are greatly reduced. Several studies have shown good maintenance of change at follow-up, ranging from 6 months to 6 years.

Interpersonal psychotherapy (IPT) was initially developed as a brief treatment for depression and anxiety problems in adults. The idea is that emotional problems are best conceived of as a result of interpersonal problems, particularly current ones. Treatment for bulimia using IPT also focuses on the interpersonal context within which the eating disorder developed and is maintained, with the aim of helping the patient make specific changes in identified interpersonal problem areas. So, in direct distinction from CBT, the focus is not on changing behaviors or cognitions related directly to bulimia. In fact, little attention is paid to eating habits or attitudes toward weight and shape. Several studies now provide empirical support for the use of IPT to treat bulimia, though none have shown it to be superior to CBT.

Both CBT and IPT can probably be helpful to adolescents with bulimia, but we have found it important to include parents in these treatments. When they are included in treatment, parents can provide support and encouragement as well as direct assistance in helping to change bulimic behaviors and attitudes.

Nutritional Counseling

Another approach commonly used is nutritional counseling. Nutritionists have long played a role in the treatment of eating disorders, on the assumption that their expertise in diets and health can help patients reevaluate their choices along more reasonable guidelines. Usual nutritional counseling consists of providing meal plans, caloric recommendations, discussion of alternative food choices to meet nutritional requirements, and support for continued progress in making healthier food choices. To date, however, the few studies that have examined these issues have been conducted with adult patients and have found that other psychological treatments (family therapy and individual therapy) are superior to nutritional counseling. However, it may be helpful at times to consult with a nutritionist for guidance on specific nutritional requirements or difficulties.

In summary, the research literature suggests that two forms of outpatient psychotherapy may be effective for anorexia: family therapy based on the Maudsley approach and EOIT as developed by Robin and colleagues. Up to this point, family treatment has received greater attention and has more evidence to support it. However, the tradition of psychodynamic psychotherapy lends additional credibility to EOIT. For bulimia nervosa, although no treatment studies for adolescents have been completed, the best evidence suggests that CBT is the treatment of choice. As noted, it is likely that this approach needs to be modified for adolescents to account for developmental variables in the younger group, specifically, with the inclusion of a family component. IPT is also a likely effective treatment for bulimia, and as it has been shown to be helpful for teenagers with depression, it's a reasonable option to consider. Again, though, family involvement is usually crucial to work with adolescents in IPT. The role of nutritional counseling remains uncertain from a research perspective, though this treatment alone appears to be inadequate for most patients. Integrated into other psychological interventions, however, nutritional counseling may still have a role.

Psychiatric Medications

In addition to psychological outpatient treatments, a variety of medications have been studied to see if they are of benefit for eating disorders. Although psychotropic medications—medications that are exclusively developed for the treatment of psychiatric illnesses—can be helpful for some, it's important to appreciate how little we know about the efficacy of medications in the treatment of eating disorders.

Antidepressant and antianxiety medications have been examined in adults with anorexia and found to be of limited help, especially during periods when these patients were acutely medically compromised. Many earlier, smaller studies have demonstrated few significant improvements in patients as a result of psychopharmacological intervention. The role of medications in adolescents with anorexia has received almost no attention. Among adult patients, medications that have been prescribed most frequently include antidepressants, designed to help patients with mood problems, and low-dose neuroleptics, used to address severe obsessional thinking, psychotic-like thinking, and severe anxiety. There is little research evidence of any benefit to those with anorexia from such medications, and these medications have been shown to pose problems in that some patients report binge eating while taking them.

Studies over the last few decades have explored the role of selective serotonin reuptake inhibitors (SSRIs, such as Prozac) in the treatment of anorexia. Prozac has been tried in inpatient and outpatient settings as a means of preventing relapse in patients who have made progress in treatment. So far, findings are mostly inconclusive, and large systematic studies are not yet available. Overall, the conclusion you should draw from this limited work is that the benefits of medication in the treatment of anorexia remain quite uncertain. In fact, most clinicians will agree that *the best medicine for anorexia remains food at a dose of three meals and three snacks per day!*

Yet, please keep in mind that several other psychiatric illnesses, such as depression and anxiety, may co-occur with anorexia, as discussed in Chapter 4. If your child has such a co-occurring disorder, she may very well benefit from a course of antidepressant or antianxiety medication, as long as the medication is prescribed for the depression or the anxiety. In addition, there are a host of medical complications for anorexia, as we have elaborated on earlier, and many patients benefit from several nonpsychotropic medications that your pediatrician can prescribe to deal with abdominal discomfort or any other medical complication associated with your child's illness.

In contrast to these discouraging findings about the help medications might offer for anorexia, most studies show convincing evidence that supports the use of antidepressant medications for adults with bulimia. Researchers were prompted to pursue the use of these medications precisely because so many patients with bulimia also prove to be suffering from depression when they consult their doctors. Inasmuch as antidepressant medications are helpful in depression, they may also be helpful in bulimia. These observations led to a series of double-blind, placebo-controlled trials of antidepressants among adult patients with bulimia. In such a trial, neither the researchers nor the study participants know whether they are taking the medication under investigation or the placebo (sugar pill). Most classes of antidepressant medications have been tested in these studies, including the tricyclics, monoamine oxidase inhibitors (MAOIs), SSRIs, and atypical antidepressants such as bupropion and trazodone. In almost all these studies, both tricyclics and fluoxetine (the SSRI most commonly known by the trade name Prozac) have proven to be better than the placebo in terms of the reduction in binge frequency. Generally, depression and preoccupation with shape and weight also show greater improvement with medication as opposed to placebo pills. Overall response to medication treatment alone for bulimia nervosa is less than for psychological treatment alone.

Perhaps the most important finding is that there is little evidence for the long-term effect of pharmacological treatment. Only one group of researchers has shown that 6 months of treatment with desipramine, an antidepressant, produced lasting improvement even after the medication was withdrawn.

Several controlled studies have looked at medication *and* psychotherapy treatments for bulimia in adults. These studies evaluated the relative (medication vs. psychotherapy) as well as the combined (medication plus psychotherapy) effectiveness of CBT and antidepressant drug treatment. These studies indicate that (1) CBT is superior to medication alone, (2) combining CBT with medication is significantly more effective than medication alone, and (3) combining CBT and medication provides only modest incremental benefits over CBT alone. The result is that patients who receive CBT versus medication are often less likely to drop out of treatment. A recent meta-analysis (combining data from several studies to increase statistical significance) of psychosocial and pharmacological treatment studies for adult bulimia confirmed CBT as the treatment of choice. Taken together, these outcomes mean that *just* receiving antidepressant medication is seldom sufficient. So when medications are used, other psychological treatments (e.g., CBT) should almost always

be included. Another finding that favors CBT is that psychotherapies are usually more acceptable to patients as compared with
medication.

In summary, recent studies of treatment for adults with
bulimia have demonstrated that CBT and antidepressant medications (especially SSRIs such as Prozac) are potentially effective
treatments. No treatment study that exclusively involves adolescents with bulimia has been published, however. Until adolescents are studied, whether treatments that have shown to be
helpful for adults can be applied to adolescents is speculative.
However, many adolescents do benefit from the same medications that have been tested in adult populations. As a parent, you
might want to make sure that your doctor appreciates this fact
and exercises the necessary caution when prescribing medications. Even if these treatments can be applied to adolescents, we
do not know whether they are as effective for adolescents as for
adults. You should therefore carefully question your doctor in
terms of how she might apply these findings gathered from
adults with bulimia to your adolescent.

INTENSIVE TREATMENTS

Unfortunately, a significant minority of those with anorexia, and
many with bulimia, who are critically ill may require a period of
inpatient treatment. Inpatient, day-patient, and residential treatments all have one thing in common: Your child receives treatment at a health care facility, either full-time or for a large portion of each day. This usually means that you will not be involved
in the day-to-day management of your child's eating problems,
although the treatment team may work with you to varying
degrees, depending on the therapeutic approach of the facility.
In this section we discuss the scientific support available that suggests that intensive treatments such as inpatient hospital programs are helpful for eating disorders.

Many parents we've counseled have expressed confusion
about the differences between inpatient, day-patient, and residential treatments. Inpatient treatment is usually indicated when
someone is in urgent need of weight restoration or has other

acute medical problems associated with an eating disorder. Once these problems are addressed, many patients are transferred to a day-patient program. Here the patient is further encouraged to gain weight and eliminate other disordered eating behaviors, but gets to go home every evening and weekend. Finally, residential treatment looks a lot like an inpatient program but usually seems to serve the purpose of accommodating those patients who may have a "failed" other treatments and require quite a lengthy stay (up to several months) to help them get back on track. In essence, though, there are perhaps more similarities than differences between these three intensive treatment approaches.

All three forms of intensive treatment attempt to, first, restore weight and stop or significantly decrease binge eating and purging, if these are concerns. Second, the programs aim to help the patients learn to manage continuing health on their own and assist the patients through a variety of forms of psychotherapy to reach an improved understanding of why they developed an eating disorder or are maintaining one. All the while, the patients are supported and encouraged through psychotherapeutic meetings in a group format and, often, in family therapy settings as well.

However, in addition to providing psychological insight-oriented therapies, it's fair to say that many such programs follow a behavioral approach. What this means (again, whether in an inpatient, day-patient, or residential setting) is that a primary focus of day-to-day activity will be centered on eating and disordered eating behaviors. In practice, this means that for those who are severely underweight, independence will initially be restricted so as to conserve energy; as they gain weight, they will also be released from the restriction of bed rest or may start participating in a supervised but limited exercise program. For those with unremitting binge eating or purging or over-exercising, close observation by professional staff is designed to prevent those behaviors with the idea that disrupting the chronic practice of these behaviors will help to reduce their recurrence. Overall, these prohibitions and observations by professional staff are decreased as the patient demonstrates improvement. The idea is that you gain greater freedom, in terms of both independence and food decisions, as you return to normal weight and eating behaviors. These activities take place in all three of these treatment settings, with the difference often being the length of stay and the number of hours spent in the treatment setting from day to day, as well as the extent to which and speed at which independence is encouraged and permitted.

Several investigators have published reports on the effectiveness of hospitalization in the treatment of anorexia, but there are no comparable studies for bulimia. In most cases, specialist units are quite successful at refeeding patients and restoring a healthy body weight. For example, one study found overall clinical improvement in the 16 participating patients after an average of 3 months of inpatient treatment using a behavioral approach, whereby the patient gains more freedom/rewards as weight increases. Also, using a behavioral approach, another researcher found that 70% of patients showed continued improvement at 3-year follow-up when treated for a period of 6 months as inpatients. These studies together indicate that inpatient treatment is likely to result in clinical improvement. It's important to keep in mind, though, that what happens in study settings is often very different from what happens in reality. For instance, a study protocol may allow for relatively lengthy treatment stays, whereas in practice you may find that your insurance company will pay for only a few weeks of treatment.

One of the discouraging aspects of inpatient treatment is that within a few short weeks of discharge many patients promptly lose the weight they painstakingly gained, even when they have had months of intensive treatment. For instance, one researcher who reviewed inpatient treatments reported that at least 40% of hospitalized patients are readmitted at least once. Further, this report indicates that eating-disordered patients spent *more* time in the hospital with each succeeding admission than any other patient group with nonorganic disorders. In other words, many patients, especially those with anorexia, seem to spend an inordinate amount of their young lives in hospitals. We've pointed out that for many patients inpatient stays are, unfortunately, necessary. For adolescents, in particular, we try to limit this time away from family and friends as much as possible.

WHAT CONCLUSIONS SHOULD YOU DRAW
ABOUT THE TREATMENTS AVAILABLE
FOR EATING DISORDERS?

The results from the empirical data so far available about all the treatments reviewed in this chapter fall within the modest-to-moderate range, and treatment studies to date are few. Still, several clear guidelines have emerged from these studies, as well as from our own experience with patients.

First, it's of paramount importance that you act early when your child shows signs of an eating disorder. Please don't hesitate or worry that you'll be seen as overreacting or interfering. Detecting and treating any illness in its early stages is invariably more favorable than waiting for the symptoms to set in and become more intractable.

Next, your involvement, especially in outpatient treatments, should be the rule and not the exception. Although you may feel ill equipped to tackle an illness as severe as an eating disorder, this concern is usually unfounded. Eating disorders are complex illnesses, and successful treatment often requires the dedicated efforts of a team of professionals (psychologists, psychiatrists, pediatricians, nutritionists). Each of these professionals will help with your adolescent's treatment program, and each will address an important part of the problem. You should be able to count on the expertise of these professionals, but they should also recognize the important contribution you can make. No matter how your child came to have an eating disorder, as a parent you know your child best and you spend more time with your son or daughter than any of the professionals on the treatment team. You not only have a lot to offer; your participation is critical because your teenager will be under your supervision more than anyone else's.

Third, early and careful attention to medical problems associated with eating disorders is critical. Too often, energetic attempts at addressing the causes of the illness are pursued prior to taking care of the life-threatening symptoms of an eating disorder. If your parental instinct tells you your child is in trouble, but the professional you consult wants to explore why your daughter won't eat or your son is throwing up his dinner every night, insist on immediate attention to the urgent problem at hand: restoring your child's health. If you and the practitioner can't agree on that course of action, you need to find another expert (see Chapter 10). Most clinicians will, of course, have your teenager's best interests at heart and should be willing to work with you in returning your child to health. In the next two chapters, we discuss just how you can make sure that you're productively involved in your child's treatment, regardless of the specific treatment received.

FOR MORE INFORMATION:

Andersen, A., W. Bowers, and K. Evans, Inpatient Treatment of Anorexia Nervosa, in D. M. Garner and P. E. Garfinkel, Editors, *Handbook of Treatment for Eating Disorders*, Second Edition, 1997. New York: Guilford Press, pp. 327–353.

Attia, E., C. Haiman, B. T. Walsh, and S. R. Flater, Does Fluoxetine Augment the Inpatient Treatment of Anorexia Nervosa? *American Journal of Psychiatry*, 1998, *152*, 1070–1072.

Beumont, P., C. Beumont, S. Touyz, and H. Williams, Nutritional Counseling and Supervised Exercise, in D. M. Garner and P. E. Garfinkel, Editors, *Handbook of Treatment for Eating Disorders*, Second Edition, 1997. New York: Guilford Press, pp. 178–187.

Garfinkel, P., and B. T. Walsh, Drug Therapies, in D. M. Garner and P. E. Garfinkel, Editors, *Handbook of Treatment for Eating Disorders*, Second Edition, 1997. New York: Guilford Press, pp. 372–382.

Kaplan, A., and M. Olmsted, Partial Hospitalization, in D. M. Garner and P. E. Garfinkel, Editors, *Handbook of Treatment for Eating Disorders*, Second Edition, 1997. New York: Guilford Press, pp. 354–360.

Robinson, P., Day Treatments, in J. Treasure, U. Schmidt, and E. van Furth, Editors, *Handbook of Eating Disorders*, 2003. Chichester: Wiley, pp. 333–348.

Touyz, S., and P. Beumont, Behavioral Treatment to Promote Weight Gain in Anorexia Nervosa, in D. M. Garner and P. E. Garfinkel, Editors, *Handbook of Treatment for Eating Disorders*, Second Edition, 1997. New York: Guilford Press, pp. 361–371.

PART III

Making Treatment Work

HOW TO SOLVE EVERYDAY PROBLEMS TO HELP YOUR CHILD RECOVER

CHAPTER 7

TAKING CHARGE OF CHANGE
How to Apply the Family Approach to Treating Eating Disorders

"We've tried everything. We tried letting her decide. We tried to force her to eat. We threatened her. We've punished her. Nothing works."

This is what we typically hear from parents who have just been told they will be taking direct responsibility for getting their child to return to normal eating patterns. If you're involved in a form of treatment that asks you to take charge of normalizing eating behavior for your adolescent—such as family therapy as devised by the Maudsley group—you may initially be perplexed and doubtful and perhaps even frustrated by the request. Parents tell us they don't know *how* to get their son or daughter to eat—either enough or regularly. Naturally, this is a source of exasperation and increasing frustration for them. It can also feel as if the situation is creating a great rift between the parents and the child who doesn't want to eat or who wants to purge. Many parents end up feeling as if they're fighting not just this illness but the child they're trying desperately to help as well.

In this chapter and the next we discuss the range of ways you can become practically involved in helping your adolescent with various problems related to eating disorders. This chapter focuses on the family-oriented treatment approach, which informs much of this book's basic premise, wherein you are asked to be *directly responsible* for changing eating-related behaviors at home. If your daughter or son is receiving a different kind of treatment that does not ask you to take this responsibility—or even discourages it—you can and should still be involved in your child's return to health; you'll find suggestions on how to do so within the other forms of therapy used for eating disorders (described in Chapter 6) in Chapter 8.

Whether the abnormal eating pattern is related to anorexia or bulimia, you will be surprised by how successful you can be in helping your child without resorting to threats, punishments, or berating. The leverage you have as parents that no one else has is your love and commitment to your children. This is powerful leverage.

You are naturally anxious about your child's health and welfare, and this may make you unsure about what to do. A certain degree of anxiety is a good thing—it helps propel you to action—but too much anxiety can overwhelm and immobilize you. There is no denying that finding ways to help your child eat normally is challenging. You may try things that don't work well. For example, some parents try to "sneak" butter or other fat into foods. This sounds like a good idea from a nutritional perspective, but it usually leads to the child's distrusting you. We have found it better to be very clear and specific about expectations as well as very direct in stating them. This is just one example of the principles we can offer to guide you in coming up with your own ways to help your teenager begin to eat healthily again. Throughout this chapter our goal will be to help you gain confidence in your ability to handle this problem, as you have handled so many other dilemmas of parenthood, thereby alleviating anxiety.

Excessive anxiety only makes parents hesitant, which leads to another problem. Your lack of confidence and uncertainty will often be perceived as a lack of resolve. This encourages your child to resist you even more because of the hold the eating disorder has on him or her. As we said in Chapter 1, don't hesitate. Act now.

A FEW FUNDAMENTAL PRINCIPLES

As with many behavioral problems in children, some fundamental guidelines will apply here. First, come up with an approach to helping your child eat normally that you can carry out. It's not much help to say you will eat all meals with your son if you're working all day and can't possibly be there. Second, be reasonable in your expectations of both yourself and your child for making behavior changes. Changing behaviors will take some time; prepare to be patient. Third, use strategies that respect your child, but guard against succumbing to pressures to let up on your expectations. This means remembering that your child has an illness and is not fully in control of her thinking and actions. In addition, it means being sympathetic and caring rather than critical and punishing. Fourth, make sure you have support, both from other family members and friends and from professionals, because this is going to be difficult at times. If the challenge were not difficult, this kind of action on your part would not be warranted to begin with. Finally, make sure you don't give up too soon. Sometimes early success leads to lowering your guard too soon, allowing the eating problem to resurface.

When you're involved in a Maudsley-type treatment, the following specific principles will apply:

1. Work with experts who know how to help you.
2. Work together as a family.
3. Don't blame your child or yourself for the problems you're having. Blame the illness.
4. Focus on the problem before you.
5. Don't debate with your child about eating- or weight-related concerns.
6. Know when to begin backing off.
7. Take care of yourself. You are your child's best hope.

The rest of this chapter is dedicated to examining each of these principles in turn. To illustrate, we describe the experiences of many of the families we've helped treat, in addition to following 15-year-old Cindy, as she and her family take up the challenge of fighting anorexia nervosa together, throughout the chapter.

> Cindy was a very focused teenager. Her father, Bill, was an accountant, and her mother, Susan, was a real estate agent. She also had a 17-year-old brother, Todd, who attended the same high school. Cindy had always been an excellent student, though she was also somewhat shy socially. She began dieting when she was a freshman because she felt she could "improve" herself if she was more fit and healthy. As she lost weight, some girlfriends commented that she looked "really good," and this made Cindy feel more accepted and liked. However, in a few months Cindy's parents became alarmed at her weight loss. She now weighed 80 pounds at a height of 5 feet even. When her parents took her to her pediatrician, she referred Cindy and her parents to a family therapist, who used family treatment that asked Bill and Susan to take initial responsibility for refeeding Cindy.

WORK WITH EXPERTS WHO KNOW
HOW TO HELP YOU

We discussed the importance of expert evaluation and treatment in Chapter 1. This is particularly important if you're going to be in charge of directly changing eating-disordered behaviors in your home. By now you know that understanding eating disorders is not a simple matter. So, the more experience your expert has had in helping families with these problems, the deeper his or her understanding of the complexities of these disorders. And the deeper the expert's understanding, the more assistance you're likely to receive in refining your own understanding of why you may be having difficulty changing your child's eating-related behavior.

Although we strongly believe you have the skills to help your son or daughter with an eating disorder, applying those skills effectively usually requires help. An expert consults with you about what you're doing and advises you to examine what works and doesn't work. An expert with a great deal of experience can offer advice on how to improve your current efforts or what to consider when you feel you've hit a brick wall.

At the same time, an expert can help you better understand your child's thinking. This is important, because at first it will appear to your child that the therapist is "on your side" and against him or her. By helping you better understand the illness, the therapist demonstrates an understanding of your child's experience to the child, inspiring greater trust and cooperation with treatment over time.

The expert therapist will also understand that every family is different and has its own style of self-management and problem solving. An experienced therapist will be able to identify the common threads that tie together all families struggling with eating disorders without imposing one-size-fits-all recommendations. The details regarding a therapist's former patients and the examples we offer in this chapter won't necessarily be completely transferable to your own family. That's where your therapist comes in. He or she is there to help you make these principles pertinent and particular to your family.

WORK TOGETHER AS A FAMILY

In our experience parents have indeed tried many things in their efforts to help their son or daughter change the self-destructive eating patterns of anorexia or bulimia; usually, however, they haven't tried any of them consistently, confidently, and with clear commitment from both parents (see Chapter 9).

After their first family therapy meeting, Bill and Susan, parents of Cindy, felt overwhelmed and bewildered. The therapist had told them to find a way to make Cindy eat. Bill sat down with Cindy and asked her what she would eat. Cindy said she would eat her rice and steamed vegetables. Susan said she wanted her to eat a piece of chicken. Cindy refused.

Susan told her she must eat it. This led to a shouting match that ended when Cindy left the table without eating anything.

When Cindy's therapist met with the family next, she listened carefully to what had happened. First, she asked her parents if the two of them agreed that Cindy needed to eat the chicken as well as the rice and vegetables. They agreed about that. However, Bill said he couldn't stand all the yelling that went on and was happy to see Cindy eat anything. It was apparent to the therapist that although Bill and Susan agreed about what should be done, they did not have the same threshold for what that meant. The therapist explained that it was just this kind of "gap" in the plan that allowed the eating disorder to slip through and reduce their effectiveness. The therapist suggested that Susan and Bill work together to refine their plan to include what the threshold for eating enough would be and what they would do to enforce it.

The next day Bill and Susan went out for coffee. They agreed that Cindy had to eat chicken in addition to rice and vegetables. They also agreed that she would need to eat one breast, but they would allow her to choose how it should be prepared. They, not she, would prepare it, however.

What Bill and Susan did was take a *first step* toward identifying a solution to breaking the hold anorexia had on Cindy. There would be many more steps in their struggle. There are many ways that parents can *seem* to be working together, but when push comes to shove, they are not. Often they can even be working at cross purposes. This is so common we've devoted an entire chapter to it (Chapter 9). For now, though, it's important to realize how critical it is that you and your child's other parent or any other adult in the household present a united front in trying to reestablish normal eating behavior. For example, Dinah's mother diligently made her eat her meals, but her father, who believed that allowing Dinah to exercise would help motivate her to eat, took her running or to the gym most nights, effectively undermining any weight gain as she used up more calories with this exercise than she took in. Neither of these parents was "wrong," but because they didn't connect the two parts of the plan, they were not successful in working together.

> Nora's mother resented doing any direct refeeding and was angry about it, though she professed to her husband that she was behind the effort. Nora's mother would "be around" during mealtimes but did not really observe to see if Nora was actually eating. Nora knew this and easily slipped most of her food into the trash. Thus, it appeared to everyone that Nora's lack of progress was inexplicable.

Again, neither of Nora's parents was wrong. They just hadn't really agreed to the treatment approach. It turned out that Nora's mother felt that her husband had bullied her into this kind of treatment and she had not wished to confront him directly.

> Tammy's father had abandoned the family when she was just a baby. There was no other extended family nearby either, so Tammy and her mother were very close. In the case of Tammy's mother, the conflict was with herself. On one hand, she felt she had to keep her daughter from purging every day, but on the other, she felt so terrible about "watching and controlling" her teenage daughter that she found herself giving in and "ignoring" the obvious signs that Tammy was purging.

Tammy's mother's mixed impulses are very understandable. As we've discussed, the person with an eating disorder often demonstrates perfectly normal thinking in most settings—except where food and weight are concerned. Parents have described mealtimes as similar to watching a "fog" roll over their child's personality and thinking. The teenager appears perfectly normal, but when expected to consume food the parents have designated appropriate, anger, resentment, and bizarre behaviors emerge. It's very confusing to see your child thinking and acting rationally and then becoming irrational, highly emotional, or withdrawn at mealtime. This confusion may lead to uncertainty and ambivalence about your efforts to refeed your child or prevent binge eating and purging. Like Tammy's mother, you may end up hesitant to do what you need to do. Unfortunately, hesitancy leaves room for eating-disordered thinking to slip through and establish a firmer foothold, as we mentioned earlier. Feelings like those Tammy's mother experienced undermine the success of either taking control and intervening or identifying a different treatment approach (see the next chapter) that might be more consistent with a strong dislike of monitoring the child with the eating disorder.

Don't Exclude Siblings

Your other children are another resource that can help defeat eating disorders. Your own brothers and sisters are the people that you will likely have the longest relationship with in your life, and this is just as true for your child. Whether they show it or not, siblings are usually affected when one of their own has an eating disorder. They are sometimes aware of the problem before you are. However, they often feel confused, burdened by a mixed obligation to both protect and help their sibling. They can also be angry at the brother or sister with an eating disorder for "causing all these problems" for the family.

In therapy, siblings can help *support* your son or daughter with an eating disorder. First, just by coming to treatment, siblings express their interest and concern. True, at first they may come only because you force them to. However, over time they also benefit from seeing how the family together can be a resource in overcoming a problem, in this case an eating disorder. Younger siblings, ages 5–6, may not understand all that is going on, but the therapist will ask them to do something kind for their sister or brother—such as make a card or do a chore that would ordinarily be done by that sibling. Older siblings may take their brother or sister on an outing to help distract their sibling from feeling miserable about eating and gaining weight or to prevent the sibling from purging. In these ways, and many others, siblings can help make the process of changing problematic eating behaviors in the home easier.

Of course, at times siblings can be unhelpful. Monica and Delphine were twins who had always competed with one another. When Monica began to diet and lost a little weight, Delphine had to take it further. When Delphine developed anorexia, Monica was anything but supportive. She felt she had to be an "even better anorexic" than her sister. In this instance the continued competition over weight and appearance made it impossible to see the whole family together. Instead, the therapist worked with just the parents and supported each daughter separately while the parents worked to help both of them. Sometimes, brothers can continue to be insulting about weight and ridicule their sisters, though they usually learn to stop. It's helpful to understand what really lies behind these behaviors. Is it jealousy? Fear or worry? Or is it evidence of an unsalvageable relationship? Your therapist should help you figure out what's behind the behavior and how best to deal with it. In any event, as a parent, you need to act to stop this type of behavior because it will undermine your success.

DON'T BLAME YOUR CHILD OR YOURSELF

It's very difficult not to hold your son or daughter responsible when what you see before you is a child who appears to be obstinately refusing to eat. However, just as we know it's not helpful for you to feel blamed for causing an eating disorder (see Chapter 3), it is clearly also not helpful to blame your child. Remembering that your child has a life-threatening illness that distorts her thinking and experience about her weight and shape can sometimes keep your own thinking clearer about the situation. Still, this is tricky, because, of course, your child is there in front of you, and it is her voice saying "no" and her refusal to adhere to reasonable eating behaviors that is causing the problem. However, she is also clearly miserable and cannot please you or herself in this dilemma. To explain this further, let's return to Cindy's family.

At their next meeting Cindy's parents complained to the therapist about how much resistance to eating Cindy was putting up and how angry they were at her. The therapist expressed sympathy for the difficulty they were having but reminded them, by drawing on the board a Venn diagram of intersecting circles, like the one in Chapter 2, just how differently Cindy was seeing the world through the lens of anorexia nervosa. Then she reminded them that it usually wasn't helpful to blame Cindy for her preoccupation with weight loss. She had an illness that kept her from seeing things the same way others did. The therapist helped the family see how much her anorexia was overshadowing who Cindy really was—she couldn't participate in her school or social life, all her time was spent on worrying about her weight and food, and she had completely lost her sense of humor. However, the therapist noted that understanding her plight was one thing, but allowing starvation to continue was another. She once again charged them with finding a way to help Cindy eat and fight anorexia. Keeping the illness separate from Cindy was more difficult than it seemed. This was hard on Susan, who still struggled to stop seeing Cindy's eating disorder as "willful," but she would try. Bill also agreed that no matter how hard it was to listen to Cindy's wailing, he would not leave the room.

When dinnertime came, Susan and Bill put the meat they expected Cindy to eat on her plate. Cindy immediately got up and left the table. Calmly, they followed her to her room, brought her dinner with them, and sat next to her on the bed. They gently explained that they knew this was hard on her, they loved her, and they would be there to help her. They sat there for about an hour, and Cindy still refused to eat. Susan began to get angry, and Bill asked if perhaps she might want to take a break and come back in a minute. Susan thought this was a good idea and did so. Cindy now began to cry and claimed that her dinner was ruined. Bill explained that he would heat it up and she could eat it. Cindy ate a few bites and climbed into bed. Her parents explained that they would not give up on her and were happy she had eaten some of her dinner with them. Her mother said, "I know how hard it was for you to eat that because anorexia is so powerful. We'll keep trying."

It's important to understand that Cindy and her family were just beginning to work on her anorexia together. At this point, Bill and Susan had determined that their support and encouragement were the correct response to Cindy's minimal consumption *at this meal.* This does not mean they would allow Cindy to continue to eat too little food to regain weight or even sustain her. An important aspect of fighting an eating disorder is establishing consequences for not eating, as discussed later in this chapter. Setting consequences not only serves as an incentive for the child to eat but also gives parents another way to respond to not eating other than getting angry and falling prey to the instinct to blame the child for the illness.

It makes perfect sense to hold a healthy teenager responsible for her own behavior. It even makes sense to hold an eating-disordered adolescent responsible for behavior that has nothing to do with weight or food. But when it comes to eating and exercise patterns in a child with anorexia or bulimia, it's critical to remember to *separate the illness from the child.* No matter how rational she may sound, no matter how committed she is to her beliefs about eating and weight, your child is not really responsible for what she says and does with regard to food if she has an eating disorder. When you talk to her about these subjects, it's the eating disorder that answers you. And it's the eating disorder you should designate as your foe, never your son or daughter. Many parents naturally have trouble remembering that "No, I won't eat" is not coming from the same source as "No, I don't think I should have to have a curfew." A thorough understanding of the cognitive distortions described in Chapter 5 can, however, help you keep it clear in your mind that you're struggling with an illness rather than with your son or daughter.

Mike's father went into a tirade whenever he found evidence that his son was still throwing up. When Mike's dad got angry, he became critical and hostile and Mike felt as though he were being attacked. This led to increased efforts on Mike's part to hide the fact that he still hadn't completely stopped purging. This made it hard for his family to see the progress he was making or to see just where he was having continued difficulties. This meant they couldn't help him as effectively.

Anger can throw you off and make it harder for you to know that the illness is the problem and not your child. When helping your child eat, anger will definitely interfere with your success. Another way you can separate the illness from the child is to keep in mind that your child does not really choose to be ill, even if it appears that way. There may be little motivation to recover in the child with anorexia nervosa, but it's the illness that is so recalcitrant, rather than your child. Certainly, purging is frustrating because it appears to many people as wasteful and dirty. However, most children who purge their food feel trapped into doing so by their worries and anxieties about weight and have become caught in a chronic cycle that they don't know how to break out of. Keeping these facts in mind may help you contain your anger. It may also help if you try to remember that it's hard for your anger at the illness not to be perceived by your child as anger with her—for being willful, ungrateful, difficult, and frustrating.

Still, your anger about having to take on this problem is understandable. You certainly don't deserve this—and neither does your child. To keep your anger from either overwhelming you or being vented on your child, it's important to recognize the signs that this may be happening. You may notice that your patience is short, that you're jittery, that your tone of voice is tinged with sarcasm, or that you're irritated by things that you usually would let pass. When you find this is so, take a break. Find someone to talk to. Get away. Otherwise, your anger can undo much of the good work you've done.

As we've pointed out, there's not much evidence that you're to blame for your child's eating disorder. However, there is growing evidence that you can be part of the solution, regardless of the cause of the eating disorder, but only if you aren't feeling guilty and powerless. Feeling guilty is especially problematic when you're trying to get started. Blaming yourself leads to a lot of second-guessing and hesitation on your part, which gives the eating disorder room to maneuver and slip through.

Beatrice felt sure that her own weight struggles and dieting were the cause of the bulimia that her 15-year-old daughter was struggling with. She felt that it was duplicitous to ask her daughter to eat regularly when she herself had for so many years dieted while her weight yo-yoed.

Beatrice had a point—it probably wouldn't help for her to be dieting or worrying about her own weight when her daughter was struggling. But there was a difference. Beatrice had never developed an eating disorder, whereas her daughter had. By blaming herself and holding back on doing what she could to help her daughter, Beatrice was actually allowing bulimia to get a firmer grip on her child. Their family therapist pointed out that Beatrice was hesitating and not following through on monitoring her daughter because of guilt. This was ultimately more harmful than anything she might have done before, because now her daughter needed her help. Beatrice decided that even if she felt guilty, she would not let it interfere with helping her daughter. She found that helping her daughter actually lessened her guilt, especially as her daughter also began to respond.

FOCUS ON THE PROBLEM BEFORE YOU

As we suggested in Chapter 3, it's easy to become distracted and to be led down the primrose path if you spend a lot of time trying to figure out *why* your child developed an eating disorder. But there are many other ways to lose your way as well. Staying focused on what the problem is—disordered eating behaviors and beliefs—is challenging. To stay focused, it's imperative that you make changing disordered eating *the* priority, be available to intervene to change behaviors, establish a regular pattern of eating, and figure out ways to expand food choices, whether your child has anorexia or bulimia. At the same time, it's important to determine when it's reasonable to allow exercise, to prevent binge eating and purging, and to know when things are going well enough that you can begin to step back and hand control over eating back to your child. Let's examine each of these in turn to see how to stay focused.

Make Changing Disordered Eating Your Top Priority

To make changing disordered eating *the* priority sounds easy enough, but in practice families find this is harder than expected. In most families, plenty of distractions can and do interfere. The demands of work, household chores, needs of other family members, and so forth, frequently command attention. For example, Laura's family was torn between her needs and those of her two siblings. As parents, they felt it was unfair to pay such disproportionate attention to Laura and her problems. Well, it was unfair, but Laura was so malnourished that her life and future hung in the balance. Their therapist helped Laura's parents to accept the fact that this extra focus on Laura was necessary, but also to see that it was *time limited.*

> Thirteen-year-old Billy's father was torn between his son's needs and his demanding job. As CEO of a large corporation, Billy's father traveled out of state almost weekly. Perhaps because Billy's mother was free to stay home and help their son fight anorexia, his father continued to make work his first priority. The family's therapist quickly stepped in and made a persuasive case for the need for the whole family to make changing Billy's disordered eating the number-one priority. Billy's father was able to reschedule many of his upcoming trips and delegate his role to others in the company.

The demands of many professions can be compelling. And unlike Billy's family, many families will suffer financially when the parents take time off to help their child eat normally again. But for the sake of a child's continued survival and return to health, parents who take responsibility for their child's eating behaviors have to put that goal above all others. In addition, making this kind of intensive effort may appear costly at first, but in the long run it can prevent the need for even more expensive services like hospital or residential treatment.

It's your therapist's task to help you keep this priority in focus and in your sights. You may be tempted to stray off into other "interesting issues," such as why the eating disorder arose in the first place, or to find "unavoidable obstacles" to taking charge, but these diversions will only keep you from the work you need to do at this point—getting your child eating normally.

Be Available

By now you're undoubtedly getting the picture: You and/or your spouse will likely need to be *available* for all mealtimes and snacks to monitor eating at least for several weeks. This is a big adjustment for many parents, who have not been present for breakfast and lunch, or even dinner in some cases, sometimes for many years, because of work or school schedules. Accepting this requirement means that you will need to make adjustments to your personal and occupational lives. If the demands on your schedule seem onerous, go back to Chapter 1 and remind yourself that just because an eating disorder is a psychiatric illness does not mean that it is not serious. As we've shown, we see these illnesses as being on a par with any physical illness. They deserve to be given the same attention you would provide for a child after surgery, an accident, or another serious medical problem.

Although it was a difficult decision, Bill and Susan both took several weeks off from work to help Cindy. They discussed the pros and cons of this measure but ultimately decided that using sick leave and vacation time this way was necessary, as they now recognized how seriously ill Cindy was. Bill had a harder time at first, and his boss was less sympathetic than Susan's. Bill took some information about eating disorders and the treatment they were using to his boss. This helped her appreciate the gravity of Cindy's illness and Bill's concern, as well as his need to be away from work more.

Don't assume you won't be able to negotiate a fair arrangement with your employer. Taking a brief medical leave is a good idea, because presenting a unified front at all meals is potentially most powerful, but in practical terms you may have to compromise. Figure out how you can adjust your schedule to allow you to be present at as many meals as possible. Maybe you can both plan to be on hand at breakfast and dinner but will have to alternate days off work to be present for lunch and snack times. A common solution in two-parent families is to divide up mealtimes, but this does leave each of you to battle the problem alone at different meals. As we discuss in Chapter 9, this can create a lot of opportunities for parents to drift into doing things differently at their respective mealtimes with the child, with the result that the eating disorder spots a chance to slip through the crack in the unified front. This is why we strongly encourage you to try to figure out from the start how both of you can be there at all meals, at least for the first few weeks.

If you have to split up the task, consider things such as whether one of you is more of a "morning person" than the other; in that case the early riser could be assigned the job of making sure that breakfast is eaten. If only one of you can be available during the day, that one could go to school at snack and lunch times. Some parents have arranged for a school counselor or nurse to have lunch with their son or daughter, but this is usually appropriate only after some time has passed, once you have a plan that is generally working and you are getting sufficient cooperation from your child to try this (there is more on figuring out when you can step back at the end of this chapter).

If you don't have a spouse, it may be important to enlist the help of another adult relative. This can be effective even when two parents are available, as it was with Sarah, whose parents both worked but whose grandmother—who was the main cook in the house in any event—was available at all mealtimes.

It may seem that your just being present won't make a big difference in terms of your child's eating, but it will. Being there provides both emotional and structural support as well as encouragement to eat. Of course, this support and encouragement won't be afforded your child unless she too is present for all mealtimes. This sometimes means a leave from school or home study for several weeks, taken as a medical leave. This is often the preferred strategy, as it was in Cindy's case.

Susan asked Cindy's pediatrician to write a note that would excuse Cindy from school for several weeks because of her medical and psychiatric fragility. Because this was clearly appropriate, the pediatrician provided the note and Cindy's schoolwork was brought to her by a home teacher on a weekly basis. Cindy fought this arrangement at first, claiming she would miss too much work. Her parents pointed out that at this point her health, not her schoolwork, was the priority. Although they also supported Cindy's academic achievements, they said these would be irrelevant if she did not recover from anorexia nervosa. This plan allowed Cindy and the family to focus on eating rather than on the social and academic pressures at school.

As noted earlier, sometimes parents are able to attend school during the lunch hour or to work with the school to develop a flexible schedule for a few weeks to permit eating to take place at home. Understandably, most adolescents don't like their parents showing up at school to eat with them. It is, however, a reminder of the cost of the illness to them that they readily appreciate, so sometimes it's an additional motivation to the child to return to normal eating. Yet being at home for all meals can send a clear message about the importance of your child's health relative to academic work at this point in time, making it clear what the number-one priority is. You'll have to decide which will be a more powerful incentive for your child and help her make the needed changes.

Although this example focuses on the need for monitoring eating in the case of anorexia, it's just as important that regular eating occur for children with bulimia, as we have stressed; otherwise, they will be more likely to binge eat and then purge. So, your help in making sure that eating is monitored throughout the day is important for both anorexia and bulimia.

Besides both parents and the eating-disordered teenager, siblings and other family members living at home need to be available for meals too. Having the whole family eat together as much as possible definitely makes a difference, because that way your son or daughter knows that everyone is trying to help him or her. As parents, you help by making sure the right foods and amounts of food are prepared and eaten. Siblings help to alleviate the tension and stress of trying to eat and contribute to making mealtimes more normal. They also distract the eating-disordered child, to some extent, from thinking only about what she has to eat. They can also support her if she becomes angry or upset about your demands that she eat.

Seventeen-year-old Todd had had a relatively close relationship with his sister Cindy when they were younger, but he
was pretty busy with his own life now. He resented having to
be home for dinner at first. His coach told him he might
have to leave his basketball team if he missed too many practices, which often stretched into the dinner hour. Bill and
Susan worked hard to accommodate Todd's schedule because they thought he was important to helping Cindy. At
first Cindy ignored Todd, but when she saw that he made
such a big effort to be there, she turned to him more often
for support when she felt overwhelmed by fighting with her
parents.

Ballet lessons, soccer, and friends, among many other distractions, are likely to beckon your other children away from the
table at mealtimes, so you will have to make a strong case for
why everyone needs to be present and call on the assistance of
the therapist to support your request. We stress that this need to
be together for most meals will not last forever, but that it's
important now because a member of the family is ill and needs
everyone's help. Usually, when brothers and sisters realize the
urgency of getting their sibling to start eating normally or to stop
purging, they acquiesce. But you should still be prepared to find
ways to accommodate their needs too. One family excused their
other children from family dinners two nights during the week
and in this way helped them be more supportive and less resentful of helping their sister with anorexia. It will be up to you to
determine what's possible, keeping in mind the option of leaving
a sibling out of the plan for a while if that child is so resentful
about giving up the time or certain activities that his or her being
at the table is completely counterproductive. Even in this case,
though, you should continue to encourage all other siblings to
participate. Many eventually do come around. For example,
Darren, a 10-year-old boy whose sister Terry had anorexia, persisted in teasing and calling her names, but he started to change
his tune after his parents recognized how jealous he was of the
time they were spending with Terry and made an effort to
address his needs as well. This is a common problem, especially
with younger siblings, who initially feel anxious and slighted

because of the focus on a sibling with an eating disorder. It can be tough on parents to find a way to take care of all the needs of their children at once, but often, just spending a little focused time with the unaffected siblings helps a great deal to reduce tension and jealousy.

Also be prepared for the fact that many siblings don't want to be involved because they simply feel they don't know how to help at first. Over time, if encouraged, they usually find ways to help that fit their relationships with their sibling.

> At first, Todd was at a loss about what he could do to help. However, it soon became clearer that he didn't need to do anything dramatic. So, each week he would find something "nice" to do for Cindy. For example, he would ask her to play a video game (one of her choosing) after dinner or watch a video with her. As Cindy improved, he volunteered to go places with her and asked her to his games. This was enough for both Cindy and Todd. By being at the meals, Todd served as a comforting presence for his sister and a reminder that she had a relationship with someone, other than with her eating disorder.

Establish a Regular Pattern of Eating

Once you, your child with the eating disorder, and the rest of your family are able to be present during most meals, the next challenge is to structure those mealtimes throughout the day. Whether the disorder is anorexia nervosa or bulimia nervosa, regular mealtimes are imperative. Again, this practice may diverge widely from what you were doing before the eating disorder developed. In our busy lives, meals are increasingly quick, eaten alone and at haphazard times. In our experience of interviewing families, it is not uncommon at the beginning of treatment for families to have no set pattern for eating. What was pretty normal for many of these families when their children were quite young—three meals and two or three snacks—is no longer the case. So it may be a struggle at first to set up this mealtime structure again, but it is essential. In the case of anorexia nervosa, the body needs regular feeding to sustain itself physically. However, in addition, as many of those with the illness will tell you, if they skip eating for several hours, the desire to continue fasting increases. For those with bulimia nervosa, skipping meals entails another hazard—increasing the risk of binge eating because of increased hunger—so in both cases structured eating times promote normalizing eating patterns. In Cindy's case, Susan and Bill established regular mealtimes. Breakfast was at about 7:00 A.M., morning snack at about 10:00 A.M., lunch at noon, afternoon snack at 3:00 P.M., dinner at 6:00 P.M., and nighttime snack at 9:30 P.M.

You may face some difficulties in trying to structure eating. The main obstacles are usually conflicting schedules for work, school, and other activities of siblings or parents. One mother, a nurse who worked the night shift, requested a change of schedule for several months. A father who had a long morning commute prepared breakfast for his wife and son and then left it for them. In this way he could contribute to the morning meal even though he wasn't there. To understand the importance of a regular meal schedule, it may be helpful to remember when your child was an infant and you had to feed her at regular and close intervals to ensure her health and growth. For most parents that was an exhausting and demanding time, but it lasted for only a year or so in most cases. That's what has to happen again here. The difference is that back then she probably cried to let you know she was hungry. Now her illness keeps her from crying out.

Related to the difficulty in setting up a schedule, a common impediment is travel. Travel during the early part of treatment is not usually a good idea. Travel means a change of schedules, eating in restaurants, and often stressful social situations for your child, who may not be ready for it, as was the case with Tamara.

Tamara wanted to go to New York to visit relatives. She knew this would be hard, and she promised to eat, but when she got to New York she found that she couldn't. She didn't trust the restaurants, and she was not yet ready to eat with anyone other than her mother and father. When she returned, she had lost 6 pounds and was close to needing to be hospitalized because her heart rate had dropped perilously low.

Even a trip to Disneyland designed as a reward for progress can cause problems because such a reward, if it occurs too early, can backfire. The success that earned the trip can quickly disappear because of the limited availability of "safe foods" and "safe situations" for someone who is still early in recovery. Nonetheless, some travel may be necessary. When it is, parents have discovered that they need to be prepared by taking along a range of foods in case they find themselves in situations where the choices are not good or restaurants are too challenging. Sometimes this means an extra suitcase, but being prepared is well worth the inconvenience overall.

Once your child is starting to recover, brief trips can be a way of evaluating progress and promoting new experiments with eating that challenge the distorted assumptions about eating, food, and weight common to both anorexia and bulimia. Often a good way to start is to visit "safe" or "comfortable" local restaurants to see how eating goes in these environments.

There are rare instances, though, when traveling has been helpful even early in treatment. One family that had enormous difficulty being together because of work and school found that when they spent 2 weeks in Hawaii, they could actually be available and support their daughter for the first time. They didn't eat out much. Still, when they returned to the mainland, they saw the progress that had been made, and this helped motivate them to keep at it even when they were home.

Help Your Child to Eat More

When recovering from anorexia nervosa, in contrast to bulimia nervosa, one has to eat not only regularly but also a lot. This is usually the next challenge after you've gotten a pattern of eating established: how to increase the amount your child is eating.

Using their schedule, Bill and Susan tried to determine what they thought Cindy should eat at each meal and snack. At first they asked the therapist to "tell us" what she should eat. The therapist said she was confident they would figure out how to feed Cindy. She pointed out that Cindy's older brother, Todd, was a healthy high school senior. The therapist explained that the reason she could not "tell them" what to do was that Bill and Susan were the ones who had to carry out whatever plan they came up with. The therapist said she would be happy to advise them, based on her experience. She said sometimes parents didn't at first appreciate how much more their child with anorexia needed to eat. It was important to remember that gaining weight takes more eating than just maintaining weight.

Like Cindy's parents, you may find it a challenge to decide how much food to provide to your child with anorexia at each meal. Parents typically find themselves underestimating how much their son or daughter needs to eat. We've often heard, "How can she not be gaining weight? She's eating more than I do!" But what parents sometimes fail to see is that a person with anorexia nervosa is actually burning food extremely rapidly, and not until rather large quantities are consumed is it possible to make headway.

Getting your child to eat more when she thinks she doesn't want to is at the heart of the challenge of recovering from anorexia. There are lots of ways parent succeed, but first they must set *clear expectations*. Veronica's parents set out her complete meals and snacks, based on the amounts they thought she needed to eat to recover her weight loss. They would put the food she was to eat on her plate. She had absolutely no choice in what she ate or the amount. Her parents knew from experience that offering Veronica a choice put her in a predicament she couldn't yet resolve: to give up anorexia or keep it. Veronica did not like this, of course, but another part of her was somewhat relieved that she didn't have to decide. If they make me eat, she thought, I can't be held responsible. This would temporarily relieve the anxiety and stress she felt about eating and gaining weight.

Sarah's parents did it a little differently. They felt that Sarah could fill her plate and choose what to eat, but they also made it clear that if they thought what she chose was insufficient, they would add to it. For some parents, offering limited choices works well, as long as they are the ones who decide whether the amount is sufficient.

Of course, if just setting the right expectations and filling plates were enough, we probably would not need to write this book. In addition to providing enough food, you have to establish *clear consequences* for not eating.

> Veronica knew that if she did not eat, she would have to stay in her room on her bed, where she could read or do homework, but no other distractions would be permitted. She also knew that if she persisted in not eating, her parents would take her to the pediatrician, who would ultimately admit her to the hospital if her heart rate or her body temperature was too low, where she would have to stay until she was better. She knew that if that happened she would be made to eat there.

As we mentioned earlier when we talked about blame, setting consequences can help you avoid the trap of responding angrily to food refusal. This is why consequences should be established well ahead of time, certainly before the plate is on the table. Again, each family must decide on the best way to impose consequences. Sarah's parents decided not to impose consequences for failure to eat a certain amount at an individual meal. Instead, they would praise Sarah for what she did eat, ignore what she did not, but make it clear that they hoped she would do better. It was at the end of the day that they would make it clear to Sarah that if she didn't continue to gain weight, they would need to become stricter. This meant that they would offer fewer choices and allow less freedom.

An important factor to keep in mind about consequences is that for most families, these are really protections for the child. Viewing them this way may make it easier for you to impose them and for your child to accept them. When your child is malnourished, it may sound and feel like punishment to your daughter to have to stay in bed and rest, but when she is malnourished it is also *necessary,* to make sure she doesn't lose more weight through exertion. Similarly, keeping your son out of school may seem unfair and counterproductive, but school, though a source of accomplishment for many, is often actually stressful and adds to the burden of trying to fight the disordered thinking associated with an eating disorder.

Reasonable, productive consequences may also help you avoid harsher punishments, which are rarely helpful. Parents sometimes entertain the idea of imposing harsh punishments for not eating because eating disorders can be such frustrating illnesses. Most parents avoid resorting to such measures because they already, correctly, see their child as sensitive and generally responsive to more gentle correctives—at least in everything except eating. In most cases, even those who try harsher punishments quickly find them counterproductive, leading to a hardening of their child's resolve against their efforts to gain the child's cooperation.

After being clear about both what you expect and what will happen if your expectations aren't met, the next challenge is *sticking with it* and being doggedly persistent. This is where you must outlast the willful hold the eating disorder has on your child. Remember, you have several advantages. First, in situations where there are two parents, at least when you are working together, your combined energy can thwart the eating disorder more effectively. In this instance two against one (when the one is anorexia or bulimia) is fair play. Next, you are older and wiser and more experienced. You know your child and what makes her tick. You can use that information to slowly build motivation to fight anorexia within her. Moreover, even if your child is an adolescent, you continue to have both legal and parental authority to count on. These are no small advantages, inasmuch as they can allow you to make decisions on behalf of your child even when the teenager, because of her illness, refuses to cooperate with interventions like going to therapy or being admitted to a hospital. You also love your child, and your dedication to her welfare supplies a powerful reservoir of energy for you to call on when you're struggling.

Regardless of these advantages, though, you still will need to outlast, outmaneuver, and overcome the eating disorder. Like any plan, it is only a plan until and if it is *carried out*. This is where parents usually have the most difficulty. They want it to be easier, they want it be shorter, and sometimes they want someone else to do it. Carrying out the plan and consequences is the **work** that must be done, and there's no getting around it. Your patience, energy, and determination will all be tried. We like to remind parents that eating disorders don't develop overnight; instead, they begin, as we described in Chapter 1, insidiously and slyly. We like to remind parents that eating disorders must be defeated *one bite at a time*.

It might help if you think of carrying out the plan like weeding an overgrown garden. If at the beginning of the day you focus on how many weeds there are and how long it will take and how tiring the job is, you will have trouble getting past the first few feet. Instead, just starting to weed, pulling out weeds one by one, and focusing on that single weed that's rooted deeply, then moving on to the next, slowly but perceptibly, you will make progress. So, Julia's parents felt dismayed and defeated when they had only gotten Julia to eat two or three more bites of bland fish than she had the day before. They wanted to give up. They felt incompetent and angry. The therapist working with them encouraged them to see it another way. He said, "You have succeeded in helping Julia eat three bites she otherwise would not have. That is a great start. If she eats six bites tomorrow, that's better still. Hang in there." Treading the line between being clear about expectations and being flexible enough to find alternatives, while also not giving in to the eating disorder, is tricky business. While not completely overwhelming your child, you have to make it impossible for the eating disorder to slip through.

Over the next several days, every meal Cindy ate was an ordeal. Susan and Bill talked together after each attempt and tried to identify new ways to encourage their daughter. First they tried to bribe her: "If you eat this, we'll get you that new laptop." Cindy did eat, but she stopped again at the next meal. "It wasn't worth it," she said. Next they tried making her feel guilty. "Look how upset everyone is. Your mother can't sleep nights. We are all a wreck!" This made Cindy cry, and she tried to eat but ended up just feeling worse. What did appear to work was saying very little about eating or food. Just encouraging her to keep trying and making sure she rested and had little other stress or distractions seemed to be helpful. Little by little their patience and persistence began to show results. Cindy's resolve not to eat slowly began to crumble in the face of their loving determination.

First it was a mouthful of chicken, then a half cup of milk, but the progress was steady, and when the family met with the therapist and saw that Cindy was gaining weight, albeit slowly at first, they had their first taste of hope for many months.

You will often be told by your child that she's "too full" or her "stomach hurts" or she's "not hungry" and that she's "just eaten." In a way, each of these statements may contain a grain of truth, but they miss the point. For anorexia nervosa, eating more than usual is necessary. In the case of anorexia, food is literally medicine. Parents can, however, help their child with these complaints to a limited extent. One set of parents found that it helped their son to drink a liquid supplement rich in nutrition (proteins and essential fatty acids) as a regular part of his meals because it made him feel less full as well as reduced his discomfort after eating. It was also a rich source of calories. Other parents have found it helpful to make sure enough is eaten early in the day so they can be a little more flexible later on. Sometimes, something as simple as a heating pad or hot water bottle, a gentle neck rub, or another soothing activity helps, because it is really not the physical problem that is causing discomfort (though it seems to your child that it is), but more the emotional discomfort she feels about eating and the anxiety she has about gaining weight that's at the root of her complaints.

We often use the metaphor of "climbing a sand hill" to describe how one must proceed in this refeeding effort. When climbing a sand hill, you have to keep moving up the hill, or the loose sand will cause you to slip back down. If you keep moving up the hill at a sufficiently quick pace, you will find you can proceed, with effort, toward your destination. However, if you pause to rest, you begin to slide and may find yourself back where you started. Only when you've reached the top of hill can you rest.

Helping Your Child to Expand Food Choices

In addition to structuring eating times and helping your child eat more, it's important to help your child expand the types of foods she will eat. Children with eating disorders have often developed a very specific list of foods they feel comfortable eating. Often these foods are very low-calorie, non- or low-fat, and low-density foods. Or, as is the case with bulimia nervosa, there are foods that they crave (often candies, starches, breads), but they allow themselves only small amounts—until a binge episode occurs. In either case, the children's preoccupations with food choices are also further delimited by calorie counting, fat gram counting, weighing and measuring food, demands that they prepare all food for themselves (and sometimes others), and sometimes the use of specific cooking pots, plates, bowls, or utensils.

You will have to decide whether you want to approach this range of behaviors as one big problem area—in which case you might just decide what and how your child should eat—as you did when he was much younger. This means that you wouldn't permit calorie counting (or at least not base what was being eaten on a specific caloric amount); you would insist on fat consumption and require that a range of food be eaten. You see, unless challenged, each of these behaviors encourages the persistence of eating-disordered thinking. Counting calories means setting a constant measure (one that the "dieting" teenager will always wish to be lower) by which to evaluate eating. The same goes for fat grams, as well as measuring and weighing portions. In other words, this obsessiveness about food measurement reinforces disordered thinking about food. This is true of all food rules in general. The rules that the person with an eating disorder sets up appear at first to protect him from overeating and gaining weight, but such rules ultimately backfire and become a cage of regulations that prevent normal eating. So, when you challenge these rules, you are challenging the disordered thinking about food that underlies the disorders.

It can be argued that a full-scale assault on this disordered thinking is the best way to proceed, and it is the basis of many hospital and residential refeeding programs. Yet, you might feel, as many parents do, that you want to take a more gradual approach to changing these behaviors. Thus, you may want to start by allowing some of the food rules to persist if eating improves and weight gain is appropriate in the case of anorexia or if binge eating decreases in the case of bulimia. If you take this approach, you may experience a bit less early resistance about eating from your child, but you will be in for a longer haul.

Glenda's parents decided they would ask her to eat one new food a week. The *amount* she ate would be what she needed to continue to make progress on her weight gain, but in addition, she could choose one new food, usually a food that was one she was struggling with but in the past enjoyed, to add to her diet. In Glenda's case the first food to be added was cheese. She had always liked cheese but had become completely unwilling to eat it over the last 6 months because she was afraid of the fat it contained. Glenda's parents gave her a choice about *what* cheese she was going to start with, *but she had to choose one*. Glenda chose Parmesan cheese. She felt more comfortable with that because it was shredded and seemed less threatening (or fattening) as a result. She sprinkled only a little on her salad, but she tried it. Again, the process was slow at first, but gradually she became used to eating Parmesan cheese and was more willing to try other cheeses as well.

Another challenge, also involving a dairy product, that arises fairly frequently is drinking whole milk. Most adolescents who are malnourished refuse to drink whole milk. "Too much fat," they say. But fat is what many of them need, so getting them to switch from nonfat milk to whole milk (even if just for a time) can provide an important source of nutrition. "Pick your battles" is our usual advice to parents about food choices. Don't argue over a lettuce leaf. Argue over something that counts—fettuccine with cream sauce or steak and mashed potatoes. Whole milk may or may not be worth fighting for if your child's diet already contains enough calcium and fat. Dora's parents thought it was, and they simply didn't buy nonfat or low-fat milk. This was a switch for the family (and one that was only temporary, until Dora was better nourished). At first Dora balked, but when her parents gently but relentlessly prodded her, she gave in. In the beginning she took only a little milk on cereal, then a half cup with a snack, but in the end the part of Dora that knew she needed to drink milk to get better began to submit, and she actually slowly agreed that it was a good idea—at least until she was at a healthy weight.

Help Your Child to Limit Exercise

Exercise is a wonderful thing. However, in the minds of those with eating disorders, it can become an opportunity to express a great deal of pathology. In those with anorexia nervosa, exercise is an effective way to lose weight and to keep from gaining weight. In those with bulimia nervosa, exercise is sometimes used as a way of purging by making sure that any calories consumed are balanced by calories exercised away on a treadmill or bike.

It's often challenging to know how and when to intervene in relation to exercise. Certainly, if your child has anorexia nervosa and is underweight, exercise should generally be prohibited. This means letters to school (sometimes requiring a physician's note as well) exempting your child from physical education. Sometimes it means monitoring in-room exercising (sit-ups, jumping jacks, etc.). Again, your involvement is aimed at promoting the physical health of your child rather than allowing continued deterioration. So, as soon as your child is eating normally and out of medical danger, it's usually a good idea to allow exercising, in moderation, once again. As with eating, however, you may have to be scrupulous about this reintroduction at first, as it's very easy for your child to get carried away. Hence, it's helpful to lay out a careful plan. For example, you could allow 15 minutes of exercise a day to begin with, and if weight continues to improve, this can be increased to 30 minutes, where it should probably remain until all signs of the disorder are gone. In some cases it's helpful to allow exercise a bit earlier. Some parents have found this helps to improve appetite, support cooperation, and increase motivation for recovery. We think that this approach can indeed be helpful, but only if you and the medical professionals you are working with feel comfortable with it. Practically, this usually means that your child is continuing to show progress in regard to her eating and weight.

For those with bulimia nervosa, reasonable exercise, not in relation to overeating or binge eating, can help minimize frustration and increase tolerance for not purging. Often, purging is resorted to in lieu of exercise, because exercising is perceived as being more work and taking more time. Helping your child with bulimia nervosa to develop a reasonable, structured approach to exercise, very similar to that taken in structuring meals, can offset this perception. Sometimes joining a health club or a structured exercise program (kickboxing, karate, etc.) in which thinness is not a virtue works well (some types of dance classes, in which a slim appearance seems to matter, can backfire). You may want to help your child identify a friend to exercise with so she'll be more likely to stick with it. Depending on the nature of your relationship with your child, you may even be able to act as your child's exercise partner. Either way, your encouragement about this way of attaining and maintaining a healthy weight and body can be very beneficial for those with bulimia.

Help Your Child to Prevent Binge Eating and Purging

In addition to everything we've already said about normalizing eating, you'll need to prevent binge eating and purging when your child's problem includes these behaviors. In the case of binge eating, for example, you are primarily responsible for what foods are available and when they are available to be consumed in your home. Therefore, it helps a great deal for you to understand more about *what* foods are likely to lead to your child's binge eating. These foods vary from person to person, but it is usually pretty evident from what's missing from your cabinets which foods your child is likely to binge eat. Common examples are cereal (by the box), ice cream (by the half-gallon), and whole packages of cookies, potato chips, cheese, and jars of peanut butter. A general rule is that binge foods are typically high-calorie, high-fat, and often sweet foods—foods that dieters try hard to limit severely and that therefore represent an indulgence.

One teenager reported that her mother routinely baked a cake for dessert on Sunday. Each member of the family of four had a piece, leaving half a cake. This cake was a consistently available and desirable food to binge on each Sunday evening. Another child reported that the "stock" of large bags of potato chips and ice cream containers bought at wholesale food markets and stored in the pantry and refrigerator were a constant source of binge foods. It's perfectly understandable that you'll sometimes bake cakes or that you might be in the habit of buying food in quantity to economize. Until your child is in better control of binge eating, however, you may need to change these and similar ways of cooking and shopping. There are likely other ways in which you're supplying food that lends itself to binge eating that you might curtail for the time being.

In addition to making tempting foods available, you may be unwittingly supporting binge eating by not being present to prevent it. Many binge eaters will do so only in private because they're ashamed of the behavior. So, many teenagers who binge eat figure out the times when no one is likely to be around or when their activities will go undetected. There are usually several such times each day. One is after school between 3:00 and 6:00 P.M., and other times are late at night or very early in the morning. These times also fit nicely into the distorted eating pattern that usually accompanies bulimia, because long periods of "restricting"—all day or all night, for example—produce increased hunger and feelings of deprivation, leading, in response, to overeating during a binge. So it is very important that you become aware of the most likely periods your child will binge eat and make an effort to be available during those times to help prevent the behavior.

With bulimia nervosa, most purging follows the consumption of a lot of food, precipitated by guilt, shame, and anxiety about overeating and fear of gaining weight. Purging, like binge eating, is usually a secretive behavior. Because purging is effective only in emptying undigested food (to the limited degree that it is) only fairly soon (usually within 30 minutes) after eating, it is a considerably predictable behavior. So, if you know *when* your child has eaten, or particularly when he has binge eaten, you are in a position to know when he will try to purge. Thus, as in the case of binge eating, knowing the time purging is likely to occur will help you know when to be on the lookout and to implement strategies to prevent it.

It's also helpful to know *where* your child purges. This is not always so straightforward. Most, of course, purge into the toilet, but many also purge in the shower, into garbage bags, or into shrubbery. Purging is often governed by very specific rules—and can be done only under those conditions. For example, some people can purge only at home, others can purge only when no one is around, and others have rules about where they cannot purge, such as at school or at church. When these conditions are understood, it is much easier to prevent them from being met and thereby disallow the opportunity for purging. If your child purges only at home (not uncommon in the early stages of the illness), you have an advantage because you have a specific limited environment to monitor. Nonetheless, the conditions can change, and it's important to keep abreast of any changes in locations for purging because any change opens a potential loophole to allow the behavior to continue.

It is also important to learn about *how* your child purges. Most often this simply involves putting one's finger down the throat, stimulating a gag reflex. However, sometimes this is ineffective and other instruments, such as spoons, toothbrushes, nail files, and so forth, are used. Some adolescents learn about syrup of ipecac, which is used to cause emesis after poisoning. When used routinely to purge, however, it is associated with cardiac problems and even death. Over time, some people learn to purge without any direct stimulation. This means that it's possible to purge at any time and very surreptitiously, making the behavior more difficult to detect and disrupt. Nonetheless, knowledge of the means your child uses to purge will help you intervene, because you can look for the signs of continued purging activity (e.g., broken nails, scratches on the back of the hand resulting from teeth scratching them, etc.). If your child uses syrup of ipecac, it's essential that you remove this substance from your home or lock it up because of the danger it poses.

Remember, your child will feel compelled to purge if she believes she's overeaten (and in this sense, she has little choice about her wish). Further, she feels tremendous relief if she purges. Thus, purging is a very reinforcing, even if shameful and sometimes painful, behavior. Your job is to help her tolerate the discomfort of not purging while supplying other positive rein-forcements instead of purging, such as attention, distractions, or opportunities for other positive things to do. *To provide these alternatives, you need to talk to your child about what she thinks would be helpful.* Some parents have found playing a video game, watch-ing a movie, taking a walk, or going shopping may help to pre-vent purging when a period of binge eating has occurred.

Laxative abuse is another common way that some adoles-cents attempt to purge their foods. As we noted in Chapter 4, taking laxatives is a very dangerous way to go about this and is very ineffective in addition. The use of laxatives over the long term leads to a variety of medical problems, including severe abdominal pain, bloating, and intestinal plasticity. To be effec-tive, doses have to be increased, which can result in toxicity in some cases. Many who use laxatives report that they wish to feel "empty" and to "flatten their stomachs" rather than just get rid of food. Psychologically, emptying the gut feels like a relief as well. To help your child stop taking laxatives, keep several things in mind. Certain laxatives can be detected in blood or stool sam-ples, and your pediatrician can test for those, helping you to know whether your child is using them without your knowledge. In addition, laxatives can be expensive if used frequently, so if your child has a ready supply of cash, you should monitor spend-ing to make sure it isn't being used to purchase laxatives. How-ever, many adolescents also steal laxatives because of their cost. It is not uncommon for bulimic persons to be caught shoplifting laxatives.

Purging can also take the form of extreme exercise. After binge eating, your child may try to estimate the number of calo-ries she consumed and try to "run it off" on a treadmill or through other strenuous activities. This pattern of exercise purg-ing may not appear to be as harmful as taking laxatives or vomit-ing, but because of the stress it places on the body as well as the anxiety about "not getting all the calories worked off" and the time it takes, trying to compensate for a binge through exercise can exact a great toll. Your role in such a situation is to help your child exercise as a usual activity for health, not weight control per se, and especially not to compensate for abnormal binge eat-ing, which results from unduly restrictive dieting.

DON'T DEBATE WITH YOUR CHILD
ABOUT EATING- OR WEIGHT-RELATED CONCERNS

One of the most common problems parents face, and you probably will too, is the distorted thinking of the child with an eating disorder. You may believe that you should be able to get your child to "see reason," "be reasonable," or "see the light" or that she "will just get over it." At the start, this just doesn't happen very often (if at all). Instead, what happens is that you are often drawn into a variety of debates and struggles that are illogical from start to finish, except from the perspective of someone whose thinking is distorted with overconcern, unrealistic investment in, and anxiety about food, weight, and shape. We discussed in detail what this thinking is like in Chapter 5. However, when you're in the trenches, up against anorexia or bulimia, the problems that this thinking can cause you are no longer abstract; they are quite specific, and it's not always clear how to proceed. Examples of the difficulties you will face include obsessive weighing, food shopping, clothes shopping, the influence of friends, and the influence of the media and fashion.

Don't Permit Obsessive Weighing

Constant weighing is a common problem in many people with eating disorders. There is an obsessional quality to it, so much so that over time weighing becomes a way of assessing one's emotional state (feeling good or bad), one's self-worth (successful or a failure), and one's desirability (being likable or unlikable). Of course, a person's weight does not really define these attributes, but their association with weighing over time makes it seem so. In addition, weighing at really frequent intervals is deceptive and inaccurate. Too many other factors (what one's wearing, when one ate, time of day, recent activity, recent fluid intake) can change weights by 1–3 pounds. You will notice that your child may be momentarily reassured by a low weight, only to come crashing down a few hours later because of a "high" weight. You know her weight has not changed substantially, but that's not how it feels to your child. At the same time, it's important that weights be taken at regular intervals so that everyone knows how things are progressing. For all of these reasons, we recommend that during treatment weight be taken only once or twice a week. This may mean throwing out the bathroom scale (or hiding it). It is also useful if the professionals you work with agree on when weights will be taken and who will take them. There's nothing helpful about a child's weight going up in the pediatrician's office, down in the nutritionist's office, and being unchanged in the therapist's office. Having too many scales just leaves everyone confused.

Decide When It Is a Good Idea to Take Your Adolescent Grocery Shopping

Shopping for food when your child has an eating disorder can be a very difficult proposition. There will be a lot of rules you're supposed to follow, and these rules tend to change a lot. Still, some parents elect to take their child with them when shopping to help them buy foods that the child will agree to eat. In our experience, this is often counterproductive. The child wanders the grocery store aisles looking for something acceptable to eat (but finding very little) if she has anorexia nervosa, and feeling guilty and tempted if she has bulimia nervosa. So, early in treatment, though it is good to understand your child's likes and dislikes, it is often better to shop alone. Later, once recovery has started, involving your child in these excursions is useful as it allows you and the child to better see the progress being made in terms of comfort with food and more flexibility in her choices.

Hold Off Clothes Shopping Until Symptoms Are Decreased

Shopping for clothes, another common activity for teenagers, is best limited during the early part of treatment as well. Often, like weight, clothing sizes will serve as "markers" for emotional and social worth. A child's pride in being size 000 is as distorted as the shame in being size 20 in the context of an eating disorder. Overall, though, because the size that fits an adolescent with anorexia nervosa will be increasing, it just makes sense to wait until full (or nearly full) weight recovery before shopping for clothes. For those with bulimia nervosa, the issue is often one of sizes going up and down during the period of early treatment, meaning that here too it's better to wait.

One shopping trip you may not be able to avoid is the one for a special outfit for a dance, particularly a dress for a girl. Such dresses and occasions often stimulate much anxiety on everyone's part. Be sure to evaluate your own investment in this process inasmuch as fashion and appearance affect us all. Try to avoid dresses that are too form fitting, regardless of how stylish, because they tend to emphasize many of the characteristics, for good or ill, that your child worries so much about.

Allow Supportive Friendships

Parents often worry about whether a friend who has an eating disorder will have a negative impact on their child's progress. There is no simple answer to this question, because so much depends on the friend and your child. There are a great number of teenagers with eating disorders, so it is likely you won't be able to avoid them. If, however, your child's friend is not being treated and also appears to be encouraging eating-disordered behaviors in your child, it would be wise to limit this friendship as much as possible, at least during the early period of treatment. This is a delicate problem, though, because teenagers' friends are very important to them. If you feel it is absolutely necessary to limit contact with a particular friend, be clear about your reasons and about your intention to reevaluate the situation as your child continues and maintains progress. Certainly, an issue of this type is important to discuss with your child's therapist to get further guidance.

Limit the Influence of Media-Related Values Regarding Weight

A number of influences beyond your home and family will have an impact on how your child thinks about him- or herself. Some of these influences are general and affect all of us in one way or another (e.g., media, fashion, and culture), others are peculiar to the adolescent world (adolescent peer groups and values), and some to the world of eating disorders (pro-eating disorder websites). How can you limit the negative aspects of these external influences insofar as they may keep your child from fully recovering from an eating disorder?

Adolescents are particularly vulnerable to the influences of media productions. They are still developing a sense of who they are and are seeking outside confirmation for their emerging identities. Ironically, in a sense, adolescents often seek to conform to a set of norms as defined by the media rather than finding their own niches. This decision to conform has to do with the need to "fit in" with a peer group. Fitting in with a peer group is important for several reasons. First, as social animals, humans naturally seek out others. During adolescence relationships outside the family constitute the vehicle whereby social learning, including dating, takes place. As a result, adolescents invest highly in their peer groups. They want to be liked, and this may take on a very simple and concrete meaning for them: Being thin (or thinner) will make them more likable. It's easy to understand why adolescents see things this way—there's a certain degree of truth to this perception. However, they often fail to see that this is hardly the sole basis for being valued. Someone is more often liked because of being funny, smart, or kind. In addition, adolescents are still developing a sense of perspective. They turn to the media and their various products to help them see things outside their smaller world. Unfortunately, the popular media, on the whole, do not provide a real perspective, but instead a highly distorted one, where beauty and attractiveness define success, happiness, and accomplishment.

As a parent, it's your responsibility to help to reestablish other values. When we talk to adolescents with eating disorders, we sometimes ask them to rank the relative importance of their weight or shape as compared with other attributes or concerns. Those with eating disorders substantially overvalue their weight and shape as compared with their intelligence, personality, friends, family, and even religious beliefs. Of course, weight is important for both health and attractiveness, but when it is *so* important that it substantially outranks all these other important qualities and relationships, it becomes a problem. It's more difficult for your child to see these other values, particularly in the

visual media. The media cannot place values on these other factors—they're harder to capture in a picture for one thing—and
even if they did, these things wouldn't "sell" because they are
unfortunately not perceived as "rare" or "special" the way beauty
is.

As a parent of an adolescent, you are in a difficult position.
You are an adult, and as such you are "out of touch," as it were
(or as it seems), with the world of your teenager. If you directly
question particulars in fashion (bell bottoms, low-slung jeans,
halter tops, etc.), you will likely be dismissed. Therefore, it's
important to approach the matter with more of a questioning
attitude than a critical one. This means that if you want to help
your child consider heroes or heroines outside the celebrity
group, it's important to try to understand what other values your
child holds that you might be able to tap into to encourage her
in those directions. For example, if your child values academic
or athletic achievement, these can be supported as alternatives
to physical beauty in terms of value. It's also often possible to tap
into the altruistic sentiments of many adolescents by identifying
ways in which social values are opportunities for balancing the
relative merits of physical attractiveness and other sources of
self-esteem and self-worth, such as volunteering, tutoring, con-
servation programs, religious and church groups.

The need for parents to respond to a child's overvaluing of
appearance and attractiveness is not unique to parents whose
children have eating disorders. However, you have a special task
because your child has developed specific problems that play
into the worst aspects of the physical ideals set up to be admired.
Your mandate is to monitor and limit the influence of the values
being promoted, at the same time identifying alternative sources
and supporting your child in turning to them for the development of self-esteem and values.

Sometimes the media communicating health issues are even
more problematic than the media promoting fashion and celebrity. This is the case, in part, because it is difficult to see health as
a problematic value. What is problematic is the way health is
defined. For example, there is frequent emphasis on vegetarian-
ism, low-fat/nonfat foods, dieting, and certain kinds of intensive

exercise regimens. The problem is that in the hands (and head) of someone with an eating disorder, the worth of these things is exaggerated way out of reasonable proportion. We like to stress that most of these choices, when made in pursuit of health, lead to good outcomes, but when they are desired in order to diet or maintain an extremely low body weight, they do not.

Among the most insidious forces that now encroach on the health of adolescents with eating disorders are pro-eating disorder websites. These websites, cleverly labeled to be misleading, provide chat groups, information, and strategies that encourage adolescents to develop eating disorders, refuse intervention, and oppose parental involvement in their treatment. There is no easy solution. Free speech is guaranteed. However, as a parent you do have some options. It may seem draconian, but for the period of time that your child is in treatment, it may be necessary to disconnect his or her computer from the Internet or to allow it to be used only under very close supervision. You can learn techniques for detecting your adolescent's use of such sites—tracing "cookies"—but as is often the case, your child may be more savvy about computer use than you. Still, the perniciousness of these sites is so strong that we recommend taking a firm stance against accessing them by whatever means you have at your disposal. Of course, your adolescent may be able to access these sites from other venues (school, library, or friends), but the time he or she has will be more limited.

KNOW WHEN TO BEGIN BACKING OFF

As hard as it may be to imagine now, there will come a time when you will need to figure out how to begin backing off from being so involved in the day-to-day management of your child's eating disorder symptoms and behaviors. In fact, that is the ultimate goal of your getting so involved in the first place. You will know you're approaching that point when your child is at or very near her normal weight, is eating reasonable amounts on a reasonable schedule, is not compulsive in exercising, is not binge eating or purging, and is generally more like her old self. If your daughter lost her menstrual period, its return is also a very good indicator of physical health.

It can be difficult to let go after struggling so hard to get a hold on this problem. It's a frightening experience to see someone whose life you treasure veer off in a dangerous direction. Studies of childhood cancer survivors have shown that the kids who went through all the chemotherapy, radiation, and surgeries were, at a later point, not particularly preoccupied with those events. Yet, their parents still had many worries, intrusive thoughts, dreams, and continued anxieties about what their child went through long before. So, keep in mind that your child may move on and feel out of danger (and may even be right about this) before you feel comfortable again.

In regard to your starting to hand control back to your child, we often use the analogy of how you might manage letting your child drive again after a traffic infraction. You might start by allowing him to drive only to and from school, then later allowing him to drive in the daytime on weekends, and so on, until full privileges have been earned. With respect to eating, you might start with allowing your teenager to eat snacks unmonitored, then lunches, and so on, until you are confident that eating is going well without your supervision. This may take several months to accomplish fully. Usually, by this time, you are more comfortable and know what to look for and how to help if problems arise.

We strongly encourage you, though, to try to allow as many other social activities as possible as your child is beginning to recover. We suggest that you do this—in part, because such engagements permit more normal development—while also ensuring that eating takes place. This may mean having to schedule activities after or before mealtimes when you're first getting started. Still, by encouraging these activities, you will be able to help your child see you as controlling only her eating behaviors and not interfering as much with other age-appropriate activities. Such an approach may also help your child tolerate your involvement in the area of eating.

We like to say that the ultimate goal in treating an eating disorder is to have *life* replace the obsessional behaviors and the thoughts about food and weight associated with them. For your adolescent, this means returning to school, taking up the challenge of explaining to her friends where she's been, and slowly entering a more normal adolescent social life. Returning to school is a worry, as the need to perform at high levels is so common to many with eating disorders. Because they've been ill, they feel they are behind, less well prepared, and as if they will never achieve what they hope to. Helping a child get back to school requires, in part, accepting that some of this concern is OK. The thought to convey is, "You can still be a good student, catch up, and be successful even if you don't take five AP (advanced placement) classes in your junior year." It requires a bit more tact or judgment to decide how much about why the child has been out of school is appropriate to share. Most teenagers just say they had "heart problems" or "stomach problems" or something to that effect. Others, like Cindy, decide they want to help others through their experience. They become peer health aides who try to help other people with eating problems.

You may find that you need to help get your adolescent back on track with these things by encouraging him more actively than you might have expected to. You may sometimes even have to take the lead in arranging visits with friends and encouraging attendance at school functions. Many children with eating disorders have some degree of social anxiety. This may have to be addressed even after the eating-disordered behavior and thinking have subsided. Treatment for these problems, as for other psychiatric difficulties like depression or obsessive–compulsive disorder, may require separate treatment with medications, therapy, or both.

TAKE CARE OF YOURSELF

It was probably evident to you as you read this chapter that helping your child will be a lot of work. So it's important that while you're doing this crucial job you take care of yourself as much as possible. If you're not able to continue to support your child, she will lose her most important asset in her fight against her eating disorder. To take care of yourself, you must recognize that you will need more rest, regular exercise, and good nutrition. You should also plan on sharing the burden with your spouse and with other family members when you need a break. If you find yourself feeling depressed or overanxious, consider seeking additional personal therapy for support. In our experience, it has not been at all unusual for parents to seek such support. You may also find support through your family, friends, or spiritual community. Making use of your own support system will help both you and your child.

At the end of all this work, though, will be the great satisfaction that you have helped your child with a life-threatening problem. Although we cannot guarantee the outcome, as we have stated before, there's very good reason to be optimistic about your chances.

FOR MORE INFORMATION

Dare, C., and I. Eisler, Family Therapy for Anorexia Nervosa, in D. M. Garner and P. E. Garfinkel, Editors, *Handbook of Treatment for Eating Disorders*, Second Edition, 1997. New York: Guilford Press, pp. 307–324.

Dare, C., I. Eisler, G. Russell, and G. Szmukler, Family Therapy for Anorexia Nervosa: Implications from the Results of a Controlled Trial of Family and Individual Therapy. *Journal of Marital and Family Therapy*, 1990, *16*, 39–57.

Eisler, I., D. le Grange, and E. Asen, Family Interventions, in J. Treasure, U. Schmidt, and E. van Furth, Editors, *Handbook of Eating Disorders*, 2003. Chichester, England: Wiley, pp. 291–310.

Krautter, T., and J. Lock, Is Manualized Family-Based Treatment for Adolescent Anorexia Nervosa Acceptable to Patients? Patient Satisfaction at End of Treatment. *Journal of Family Therapy*, 2004, *26*, 65–81.

le Grange, D., and J. Lock, Bulimia Nervosa in Adolescents: Treatment, Eating Pathology, and Comorbidity. *South African Psychiatry Review*, 2002, *5*, 19–22.

le Grange, D., J. Lock, and M. Dymek, Family-Based Therapy for Adolescents with Bulimia Nervosa. *American Journal of Psychotherapy*, 2003, *67*, 237–251.

le Grange, D., K. L. Loeb, S. Van Orman, and C. C. Jellar, Bulimia Nervosa in Adolescents: A Disorder in Evolution? *Archives of Pediatrics and Adolescent Medicine*, 2004, *158*, 478–482.

Lock, J., Treating Adolescents with Eating Disorders in the Family Context: Empirical and Theoretical Considerations. *Child and Adolescent Psychiatric Clinics of North America*, 2002, *11*, 331–342.

Lock, J., D. le Grange, W. S. Agras, and C. Dare, *Treatment Manual for Anorexia Nervosa: A Family-Based Approach*, 2001. New York: Guilford Press.

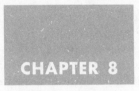

CHAPTER 8

PLAYING A SUPPORTING ROLE

Other Ways You Can Be
a Part of Your Child's Recovery

In Chapter 7 we focused on ways you can be involved in *directly* changing disordered eating and related behaviors through family therapy based on the Maudsley model. In this chapter we illustrate how you can be involved in other types of treatment as well. The treatments discussed in this chapter were not developed with the tenets of the Maudsley approach in mind, and they vary in their adaptability to parental involvement. How much you are permitted and encouraged to participate may also vary from practitioner to practitioner within the same form of therapy. But all of these therapies can be delivered in ways that do not exclude you, that show respect and support for your role as parents, that educate you about what is being done to help your child, and that specify how you *can* help. Your involvement in these other therapies is just as important as in family treatment, though your role in changing behaviors is usually more *indirect*.

In earlier chapters we stressed that the importance of parents in supporting adolescent development has been underestimated. Increasingly, it is clear that involved parents make a real difference in how successfully children and teenagers negotiate their lives. So, whether you take a direct or an indirect role in helping your child, your involvement will likely make a significant contribution to your child's recovery.

PRINCIPLES FOR PLAYING A SUPPORTING ROLE

In the following pages we discuss how you might be involved in intensive treatments (such as inpatient programs, residential programs, and day programs) as well as in outpatient psychotherapies, especially individual approaches. Your involvement in any of these forms of treatment will vary in the particulars, but there are some general principles that apply to all of them.

1. Agree on the Approach You Will Try.

As we've stressed from the outset, one of the biggest obstacles to helping your child recover is disagreement between parents about how to help. How you can address these difficulties is detailed in Chapter 9. However, even before you make the first appointment, try to get your heads together to see if you can determine where the differences are and identify the treatment that makes the most sense for your child and family.

See Chapter 6 for information on the data available on the effectiveness of each type of therapy. If you don't find the therapy you're considering in that chapter, ask the referring doctor why he or she believes that type of treatment may help and why it might be a better choice than the therapies that show the greatest effectiveness in recent, reliable research. If the doctor does not have an answer that satisfies you, and the therapy does not fall into any of the categories discussed in Chapter 6, you can be fairly sure that there is no reason to expect it to be effective in improving your child's symptoms, which means that wasting time on it could endanger your child's health needlessly. Ask for another referral, and if you don't get one, see the Resources section of this book for other ideas on finding a good source of help.

When we advise you to come to agreement on which approach to try, we mean that you should include only you and your child's other parent or guardian. Don't make your child part of this decision. It's counterproductive to allow your child to have too much say in which steps will be taken to eliminate an eating disorder because, before your child begins to recover, when you talk to her about the problem, you'll end up hearing from the disorder more than from your daughter. This doesn't mean that you cannot ask your child's opinions, but the decision remains in your hands as parents. By reading this book you are preparing yourself to make a decision on how to help your child with an eating disorder. Your child may have opinions and strong feelings about what treatment is desirable, but as you now know, motivation for recovery is not high in many adolescents with eating disorders. Ultimately, then, it will be up to you to assess the treatment options and to decide how best to proceed.

2. Learn All You Can about Any Treatment You Choose.

The introduction to the various treatment approaches for eating disorders we provide in this book is limited in scope and detail. So, as you consider the different options in more detail, you should seek out additional resources and information. Chapter 6 contains information on research evidence as of the publication of this book, but data from ongoing studies are always accumulating, so you may want to stay abreast of any results published in the interim. The Resources and Further Reading sections of this book will give you sources to consult for both types of information. Your child's pediatrician, too, may be able to tell you where you'll find reliable sources of up-to-date research, and if you are already working with a therapist, he or she may be able to provide you with handouts about various treatment approaches.

3. Share Your Perspectives on Your Child and His or Her Treatment from the Start.

As we've said, anyone who is treating your child should ask you to describe your child's development and to give your observations of the child's current behaviors and symptoms. However, you should also take the opportunity to share as much as you can about what you think are contributing problems and conflicts, as well as any strengths and abilities that may be called on in both your child and your family as a whole. Providing this information and sharing your perspectives with your therapist will allow you to begin to forge a relationship in which you are working together from the start. If you have trouble in continuing to work together, Chapter 10 has ideas for improving your teamwork.

4. Keep in Frequent Contact with any Therapists or Physicians Involved in Providing Treatment.

Sometimes parents feel that once a professional is involved, their responsibility is over. Other parents feel they cannot or should not ask a therapist questions or get feedback on how their child is doing. Neither of these is a sound perspective. Although there are some areas in which confidentiality between a teenager and his or her individual therapist should and must be respected (sexual behaviors, intimate feelings, social activities), you still need to be involved. Regardless of the approach, your perspectives on why the disorder developed, how symptoms are currently being expressed, and how you and your family are being affected by your son's or daughter's ongoing struggles are all appropriate areas for regular discussions with the therapist.

5. Determine How You Will Assess Progress.

One thing that is helpful to ask the therapist at the beginning of treatment is what to expect in terms of improvement of symptoms and over what time period. This way everyone has an agreed-upon benchmark to use that, though not ironclad, will likely help everyone see the trajectory of recovery. If you also agree on how and when you'll be updated on how things are going, you'll go a long way toward ensuring that your child is getting the treatment she or he needs at this time. This updating should be negotiated between you, the therapist, and your child to allow you to evaluate how things are going at reasonable intervals. For example, with a child who suffers from anorexia, never knowing for sure if your child is gaining weight will make it difficult for you to assess your child's progress. Also, if your child purges, but does so surreptitiously, you might not know when she's doing better or worse.

6. Have a Backup Plan.

Although one of the biggest mistakes we see parents make is to keep changing therapists and treatment approaches, we nonetheless feel that you should keep your options open in case the approach you take doesn't work for your child. No treatment for any condition works 100% of the time for everyone, so it's best to be prepared with an alternate plan should progress not be as you, your child, and the therapist had hoped. Having a backup plan is not the same as undercutting a current therapy, but rather a way of making sure you aren't caught without alternatives—because, as we've said many times throughout this book, the longer these problems persist, the harder they are to change. To make a backup plan, work together as parents with your therapist and physician to see what would be the best next step as soon as progress is definitively stalled. The treatments described in Chapter 6 should provide a good start for you in evaluating your options.

7. Keep Your Child in Treatment.

Although your role in most forms of individual therapy is somewhat circumscribed, it's still very important, partly because your child's motivation to be treated for eating problems is initially apt to be low. So you can expect that you will need to encourage, support, and even insist on your adolescent's attending treatment sessions. This may mean that you will have to work with your child's school to excuse her from classes so she can attend treatment, inasmuch as it is usually impossible for all therapy sessions to take place outside of school hours. This can cause another struggle with your child, who may not want to miss classes or time with friends. In addition, you will likely be asked to participate in some treatment sessions. The content of these sessions will vary, depending on the type of therapy your child is being provided. Regardless, make it a priority to attend these sessions. Your attendance helps to send a message that you support the treatment even if you're not the main player.

HOW YOU CAN STAY INVOLVED
EVEN WHEN YOU'RE NOT IN CHARGE

Throughout this book we have acknowledged how difficult it can be to be excluded from your child's treatment, whether you're just left uninformed or told directly to stay out of it. It's especially tough when this catches you off guard. If you don't know how you *can* participate, you'll feel pretty powerless to find a role in your child's recovery. The rest of this chapter shows specific ways you can remain involved in various forms of therapy. Even though inpatient treatment is neither the most common nor the best-studied treatment setting, it serves as a paradigm for parental participation when you're not directly in charge of treatment, as you would be in Maudsley-type family therapy, so we'll start there.

What is your role in intensive treatments (hospitals, residential programs, and day treatment programs)?

Unfortunately, many children with eating disorders need intensive treatment provided in some type of institutional setting. Depending on the goals of these programs, the term of inpatient treatment may be as short as a few days to as long as 12 weeks. When inpatient treatment is used purely to stabilize an adolescent's acute medical problems, such as when the patient needs rehydration, the stay will likely be only a few days long and probably in a pediatric medical unit rather than an eating disorders unit. When the primary goal for inpatient treatment is to restore weight and give treatment-resistant patients with life-threatening weight loss a real chance at recovery, inpatient treatment might last between 10 and 12 weeks. However, for some programs the main treatment goal is to halt rapid weight loss and just jump-start weight restoration. In these instances, rather than providing several weeks of treatment, the stay might last only 10–14 days.

What you should take from this information is that you need to be sure inpatient treatment is recommended at the right time and for the right reasons. Too often, we meet parents who have felt pressured to admit their child when they were not considered in the decision-making process. Specifically, they did not receive an adequate explanation of the necessity for this particular course of action, the goals of the admission, the anticipated length of hospitalization, and why an outpatient treatment was not considered. At other times, the converse is true, when there is pressure to keep patients out of the hospital when it is, in fact, required. Instead, the child is kept in inadequate outpatient treatment because of costs. Some parents, with the help of their doctors and considerable amounts of lobbying, have succeeded in convincing their insurance companies of the dire need for hospitalization. This route, however, is not only frustrating but also very time-consuming, especially when inpatient care is urgently required. It is best to discuss your options with your child's doctor when you are concerned about your child's weight loss.

The criteria used to recommend that your child be admitted for an eating disorder will vary from one inpatient treatment team to another, but the differences should be in nuance as opposed to substance. Both you and your child's treatment team should generally adhere to most of the following guidelines when deciding whether your child should become an inpatient for acute medical reasons (a couple of days in the case of rehydration, for instance) or for a longer-term admission for weight restoration (several weeks, as discussed earlier). General guidelines for medical hospitalization have been published by the Society for Adolescent Medicine and the American Academy of Pediatrics. The precise guidelines will have to be established by your child's pediatrician, but in general they should resemble the following:

- Severe malnutrition (less than 75% of ideal weight)
- Pulse rate less than 50 beats per minute in the day, less than 46 beats per minute at night
- Temperature less than 36.4 degrees Celsius during the day, 36.0 degrees Celsius at night

- Orthostatic (lying to standing) systolic blood pressure greater than 10 millimeters of mercury or pulse change greater than 35 beats per minute
- Irregular pulse (QTc interval greater than .44 second)
- Abnormal electrolytes (usually potassium less than 3.0 milliequivalents per liter)

The need for a child to be hospitalized almost always causes considerable worry. Parents often approach inpatient treatment with just about as much trepidation as their adolescent child. Their uncertainty is further increased because the child, wanting to stay out of the hospital, exerts pressure on them. Although parent and child may have different reasons for feeling ambivalent about inpatient treatment, it's important to keep in mind that hospitalization reflects a crisis and is therefore often experienced as traumatic and certainly disruptive.

The only way to limit the impact of hospitalization is to keep the hospitalization brief, but this decision may be entirely out of your hands. So, taking your child for inpatient treatment is no easy decision. However, even if your child is in need of longer-term inpatient treatment, but it is possible to have her admitted for only a short stay, this could be a life-saving step you might have to take.

When you're weighing the possible effectiveness of inpatient treatment for your child against that of other treatment modes, be sure to consider what kind of follow-up treatment to the inpatient stay will be available. Without proper follow-up, it's often very difficult to maintain the improvements that have been achieved while the child was an inpatient. If the specialist unit at which your child may become an inpatient is near your home, regular follow-up appointments with your child's doctors may not be very complicated. If the facility is not close by, however, is another source of follow-up care on an outpatient or day-patient basis accessible? Making sure that your child's inpatient care is complemented by good follow-up treatment should be a combined effort between you and the discharging inpatient team. Make sure the team is willing and able to help in this way before making a decision on inpatient care.

Yet perhaps the most important issue at stake is your involvement in your child's inpatient treatment. How much and in what ways you're permitted to be involved while your child is an inpatient will vary with the treatment approach taken by the team, but it's important that you avail yourself of every opportunity offered to you. This is another reason that location is important. If the specialist unit at which your child will be an inpatient is far away, participating day by day may be logistically difficult for you. Yet this participation will help lay the groundwork for you to be active in maintaining your child's gains during the follow-up period after discharge. We have already alluded to the fact that many teenagers end up returning to the hospital because they don't sustain the weight gains they have made during their hospitalizations, as Brenda's case illustrates.

Brenda was only 12 when she was first admitted to a very well known inpatient unit a couple of states away from where her family lived. There was no such facility within Brenda's home state. She progressed well in the hospital and was sent home after several weeks to "take care" of her eating by herself. Unfortunately, her parents, bewildered on the sidelines and against their own better judgment, watched Brenda lose weight promptly, and they had to make the trip across state lines once again. As with the first admission, Brenda settled down in the unit and started gaining weight. Her parents were not involved in the hospital's refeeding efforts and weren't given much feedback about how they might be able to help Brenda once she was discharged again. As before, with the encouragement of the nursing staff, Brenda did really well in terms of her eating. She was discharged after several weeks at a healthy weight, and again her parents were told that it was now "up to Brenda to take care of herself." Thirteen-year-old Brenda tried hard to cope with her anxieties about eating, but again her parents remained on the sidelines as they were instructed. Consequently, she lost all the weight she had gained in the hospital just a few weeks after returning home. By now, Brenda's parents knew the road to the inpatient unit all too well. The same scenario was repeated once more.

Obviously, everyone interested in Brenda's well-being would have liked to prevent this type of cycle. To avoid the same trap with your own child, we encourage you to learn as much as you can from the inpatient team while your child is there. Here are the kinds of opportunities to look for:

1. **Parent education meetings:** These meetings are common in most inpatient settings. They provide you with an opportunity to ask questions about anorexia and bulimia and to learn more about these illnesses from experts, who will also have some specific knowledge about your child and the situation.

2. **Observation of nursing and other professional staff:** If you observe experienced staff members doing their jobs, you may learn why and how they are successful at getting your child to eat and gain weight when you haven't been. You will likely notice that they don't argue about what should be eaten or when—these expectations are clearly established.

3. **Opportunities to try helping your child eat while she's in the hospital:** Some programs encourage parents to come in for some meals to allow them to see what their child is eating and to allow them to attempt to monitor a meal themselves.

4. **Discussions with the nutritionist:** A meeting with a nutritionist while your child is in the hospital can be helpful. A nutritionist can help you understand better how much food and what types might be most helpful for your child.

5. **Parent support groups and therapy:** Many inpatient programs have support groups for parents. These groups will help you see that your struggles are not unique and can provide a useful tonic for the feelings of isolation and shame that are common to families when they first struggle with a child with an eating disorder.

Unfortunately, too often parents are excluded, or exclude themselves, from inpatient programs. This can result in a cycle of weight gain in the inpatient setting, followed by rapid weight loss at home. Eventually, the patient is "blamed" for not wanting to change, the parents' skills are not capitalized on, and the result is that the teenager is sent away to spend several months at a residential facility, which is often hundreds of miles from her family and friends.

In addition to short-stay admissions, intensive day treatment programs may be an effective alternative to longer-term, intensive inpatient treatment for some patients with eating disorders. Day treatment is sometimes recommended for those patients who have completed intensive inpatient treatment; they then "graduate" to this step-down treatment prior to being discharged from the hospital altogether. Sometimes day treatment will be deemed appropriate for a patient without the patient's having spent time in an inpatient facility. This poses a difficult decision, for essentially the doctors are telling you and your child that she is very sick but not "sick enough" to spend 24 hours a day as an inpatient—a fine line to draw.

Day treatment is a good alternative to inpatient treatment in that there is a little less disruption of regular family life and it is easier for parents to be involved in treatment. For instance, parents get to oversee an evening snack as well as all meals on the weekend. In some ways, if the day program can really involve parents in the treatment, this is a good way in which parents and program staff can learn from each other, so that by the time the teen graduates from the day program, his or her parents are more confident that they can continue to help their child, independent of the institution.

A limitation of many residential and some inpatient and day programs is that they often do not treat younger patients (under age 14) or boys. In some instances, rightly or wrongly, residential treatment is considered a treatment of last resort. When an adolescent has spent a great deal of time in outpatient treatment, and may also have had several stays in an inpatient facility, and yet his or her illness has not responded to these treatment efforts, residential treatment is often recommended. This is not to say that every patient at such a facility has failed at prior treatments; for many patients residential treatment is the first type of program in which they participate. But it's fair to say that, as a rule, several other treatment options are explored before most doctors (or parents, for that matter) consider residential treatment. At many residential centers a program for educating parents and parent support groups are part of the overall treatment.

However, by necessity, because of distance and the cost of travel, both the scope and scale of these programs are limited. Nonetheless, if your child does need to be treated in a residential facility, try to find one that involves you as much as possible and that can provide help for you when your child is discharged home.

What is your role in general family therapy for eating disorders?

The Maudsley approach to family treatment does not focus on general family problems or processes; instead, the main focus is on how the family can help with the specific symptoms of anorexia or bulimia. In contrast, many therapists use forms of family therapy that do not focus on your changing or managing your child's symptoms. Instead, these types of family therapy try to address more general family problems because they believe that these general issues contribute to either the development or maintenance of an eating disorder. As we pointed out in Chapter 6 and elsewhere, the evidence that this idea is true is very limited, but this type of family treatment is both common and felt to be effective by many clinicians, so you may encounter it among the options available to your child.

In these forms of family therapy, the therapist tries to change a variety of general family processes. Specifically, the therapist wishes to identify and correct inappropriate alliances within the family, communication problems, avoidance of conflict, and suppression of individuation and separation among family members, particularly the adolescent with an eating disorder. When family therapists discuss "inappropriate alliances," what they mean is that from their perspective families work best when parents work together and have clear authority. Sometimes, though, a child may end up getting closer to one of the parents than the other. This kind of alliance can happen, for example, when a child is very ill, requiring a parent to focus almost all of his or her energy on the child. Such an alliance can also be encouraged if there are significant problems between the parents themselves. Regardless of their origin, these alliances can interfere with parents working together, especially in terms of getting rid of an eating disorder. A therapist will attempt to help a family redress the problems created by such alliances by first identifying them and then illustrating how they are interfering with the parents' working together.

Family therapists address "communication problems" by opening the lines of dialogue. The members of many families, unfortunately, lose the capacity even to talk to one another. This can result from many factors, among the most common of which are parental preoccupation with work or responsibilities, parental anxiety or depression, and marital discord. A specific form of communication problem is *avoidance of conflict*. Conflict avoidance goes beyond the general problems of communication to a reluctance to take on significant problems in order to "keep the peace" and "avoid fighting." Avoidance of conflict is held as a higher good than solving the problem. Avoiding conflict can, unfortunately, backfire and allow problems like eating disorders to fester and grow. Therapists help families to determine when and how and sometimes why they prefer to avoid conflict over approaching a problem directly even if it means a period of hostility.

Finally, some families appear to struggle with supporting the evolution of their child's independence during adolescence. Because of worry about what might happen to their child or what the family would be like if their child were more independent, some families appear to send a covert, and sometimes overt, message that they don't support their child's growing up and leaving the family. Addressing this problem means that families have to explore why it might be hard to have a family member grow up and leave them. Common reasons that have been identified by family therapists include fear that without the child present the family will disintegrate, that parents will be lonely, and an unrealistic fear that the child is too immature to leave home.

Your role in these forms of family treatment is to make yourselves as open and available as possible to the examination of the kinds of problems discussed here. This may be easier said than done. It's challenging for all of us to open ourselves to this kind of scrutiny. In addition, remember the principles offered at the beginning of this chapter: Make sure you understand how progress will be measured and that you have a backup plan in case you can honestly say that you've given the treatment a chance and are not satisfied that it's helping—or, always, if you see your child continue to lose weight or suffer other debilitating medical consequences of the eating disorder.

What is your role in individual psychodynamic approaches?

Clearly, the main argument of this book is that parents need to actively take charge of helping their children with eating disorders. We have stressed repeatedly that eating disorders distort thinking and behavior to such a degree that, as a parent, you are your child's best hope for making significant progress. Nonetheless, other approaches based on psychodynamic therapy have been shown to be helpful in addressing the developmental and emotional problems associated with eating disorders, even if not in addressing the behaviors themselves. In this way they share some similarities with the general family treatments we just discussed. Many clinicians have practiced these types of therapy for years with a sense of clinical success. There are many individual schools of thought that can loosely be grouped as psychodynamic, but only ego-oriented individual therapy (EOIT) has been shown to be effective in treating anorexia in adolescents (see Chapter 6). We'll use it in our example of how you can be involved in individual psychodynamic psychotherapy. EOIT grew out of ideas derived from a type of psychodynamic theory called *self-psychology*. EOIT is a psychodynamic therapy that tries to resolve developmental problems to leave the child with a strong sense of self and sustained feelings of confidence and efficacy. As it pertains to anorexia, the theory suggests that children with this disorder have difficulty with feeling assertive and independent and, as a result, confuse control over eating and weight with other psychological and emotional needs related to independence and confidence. As such, it uses the therapeutic relationship with the individual therapist as the primary vehicle for promoting change.

According to this therapeutic approach, anorexia is a self-destructive attempt to manage problems with emotional immaturity, fear, anxiety, and depression by restrictive dieting and weight loss. To find alternatives to the self-destructive strategies associated with severe dieting, patients must first learn to identify and define their emotions, both positive and negative, rather than avoid awareness of these feelings through starvation. Recovery also entails increasing their sense of effectiveness in managing problems common to adolescence, including learning to successfully separate and individuate from their family of origin. Other goals of treatment are to help the adolescent develop a healthier sense of self, her family, and the challenges of adolescence and young adulthood so that she feels stronger and more capable.

Even though the main focus of EOIT is on the child, parents are routinely involved. At the beginning of EOIT, parents are oriented to the rationale for and nature of this form of therapy. Therapists meet with parents in separate (collateral) meetings where they try to assess parental functioning and family dynamics and begin to provide parents with information on how they can help their child manage the developmental challenges that are affecting the anorexia. The therapist should explain that these sessions are designed to support the parents. Parents are educated about separation and individuation being a part of normal adolescent developmental processes and are helped to better understand that what might be regarded as normal and desirable (perfectionism, compliance) are, from the theoretical perspective of EOIT, likely part of the underlying pathology of anorexia. Parents are told that improvement may lead to increasing noncompliance and disagreements with them, as testing limits in these ways is seen as normal in the quest for greater appropriate autonomy during adolescence. At the same time, a teenager's withdrawal may seem problematic to some parents, but the therapist helps them understand that during the course of recovery, this should be expected because it too is normal adolescent behavior.

Over the course of EOIT, the therapist will meet with you to assess the degree to which you are handling your child's difficulties appropriately and offer suggestions accordingly. This may be especially necessary for the welfare of younger or less assertive patients. In addition, you will be asked about how you are handling stresses in your child's life and respecting her need for confidentiality; again, the therapist may offer suggestions to help you in these tasks. For example, the therapist can help you limit the number of extracurricular activities or tutors the child has if the child feels that either is a problem. In short, the therapist serves as your child's advocate in these collateral sessions.

To help you appreciate your child's underlying dilemmas, the therapist will try to help you by suggesting ways to understand your child's behavior and thought processes (especially as they relate to the etiology and maintenance of anorexia) without violating the confidential trust between the therapist and your child. In this regard, it's sometimes helpful for the therapist to ask you for more information about any significant life events that your child has disclosed. The therapist will explain to your child the value of sharing this information. For example, it may provide an opportunity for parents to help or to create a better support system for the child. Moreover, in the process of talking with you, the therapist may discover information (for example, that there is severe marital discord or that one parent has an eating disorder) that, with your permission, will be useful to take back to individual therapy with your child. The therapist's conveying this information may help your child take your limitations less personally and feel less devastated by them. This may be particularly the case with adolescents who are especially self-critical and who have trouble viewing their parents as imperfect.

Thus, with EOIT, your role is fundamentally to support the individual therapy designed to enhance your child's capacities for mastering her dilemmas in regard to adolescence and eating. However, as you can see, you are important in the process because you provide information, support the treatment, and open yourself to changing your own attitudes and beliefs if they interfere with your child's needs.

> Sixteen-year-old Sarah had been seeing her therapist in individual treatment, and she had gradually gained weight and stopped binge eating, though she still occasionally purged when she felt she went off her diet. However, she was increasingly surly with her mother and steadfastly ignored her father whenever he spoke to her. Sarah and her therapist discussed these issues and framed them as having to do with Sarah's wish that her parents would treat her more like her 18-year-old brother.

The therapist asked to meet with Sarah's parents to discuss their view of adolescence. Sarah's mother felt that Sarah was struggling with her because they were too much alike. Sarah's father felt that Sarah was angry because they placed restrictions on whom she could date (no one older than 17) and had a curfew (no later than 10:00 P.M. on Fridays and Saturdays and no going out on school nights).

The therapist served as an educator and advocate for Sarah in the meeting with Sarah's parents. She strove to help them understand the importance of allowing some risk taking (without going overboard) to help Sarah develop more confidence in her own judgment and ability to make appropriate choices. Specifically, they agreed to allow Sarah a trial period of dating whom she chose as long as they could meet him and to allow her to be in charge of her curfew as long as she behaved responsibly.

After several weeks, the parents were asked to return to see how things were going. Although there had been some missteps (on one occasion Sarah had stayed out very late without calling), overall her parents felt that Sarah had demonstrated to them that she was capable of being more responsible than they had expected. Further, the conflicts they had been experiencing had diminished. Over time, Sarah gave up purging on a regular basis. Her conflicts with her parents were fewer and, gradually, she was less preoccupied with her weight as she became interested in her plans for college.

What is your role in supporting CBT for bulimia?

Although cognitive-behavioral therapy (CBT) for bulimia is conceived of primarily as a treatment that takes place with your child and his or her therapist, it is reasonable to involve you in treatment as well. We know you can help improve motivation, support the attempts by the therapist and your child to change behaviors and thinking, and in many cases (though not all) be involved in meal planning and monitoring for and assisting with efforts to decrease binge eating and purging episodes. Your involvement in CBT for bulimia nervosa capitalizes on your abilities to alter your home environment to support a change in binge eating and purging, similar to what you may do in family treatment, as described in Chapter 7. However, as CBT is primarily an individual therapy, your role is somewhat different and is further delineated by the various stages of CBT.

At the start of CBT treatment you will be taught about the CBT model of bulimia and how the specific interventions (self-monitoring, behavioral experiments, problem solving, and cognitive restructuring) are helpful in treating bulimia. This helps you understand what your child will be doing and may help you to determine how you can be helpful. The first task in the first stage of CBT is to regularize the eating pattern to prevent binge-eating episodes. You may be asked to assist with providing meal-time structure (three meals and two snacks) and to help prevent binge eating by limiting access to trigger foods and prevent purging by staying with your child for a certain period of time after meals.

> Sixteen-year-old Tanika's pattern of eating was to restrict her intake all morning and through the early afternoon. Then, when she got home from school, she would begin to eat a snack, but this quickly escalated into a binge-eating episode, followed by purging. The therapist discussed with Tanika various strategies for changing her eating pattern. The one that appealed to her most was to ask her mother to eat breakfast with her and to be home after school so that she could help her avoid binge eating. This meant that her mother had to leave work early for several weeks, but her support helped to change Tanika's eating patterns enough that, after several weeks, binge eating was significantly reduced.

Self-monitoring by keeping records of foods consumed and weight is a key component of CBT, although it is sometimes challenging for adolescents because it involves both the ability to self-observe and the effort of writing down these observations. Because adolescents are typically less skillful at self-monitoring than adults, you can support your child's efforts in CBT by helping her understand the importance of completing the food records. This may mean something as simple as asking if your child has a food log sheet or just gently reminding her to complete it. Usually these records are private entries that your child makes to discuss with her therapist, but sometimes, especially with younger adolescents, it may be helpful to ask if you can help the child complete these records, at least at first. Moreover, parents sometimes keep logs of their own observations of their child's behaviors and apparent emotional states. These can be used as comparison documents for discussion with the therapist and adolescent as well.

Maureen was a 14-year-old with bulimia nervosa who repeatedly denied binge eating or purging. However, the therapist routinely checked with Maureen's parents about her behaviors, and they reported that although she had had a period without binge eating, they had once again noticed a large amount of food missing and evidence in the bathrooms that purging had resumed. The therapist asked the parents to join Maureen in a session. In this session the therapist asked the parents to share their observations and concerns. The session was not confrontational, but aimed instead at helping Maureen see that although she was minimizing her symptoms, they were still a significant problem. Maureen's mother described discovering that several boxes of cookies and pints of ice cream were missing, with no explanation for their disappearance, but said she was worried that they were too tempting for Maureen to resist. Her father, who did the cleaning in the house, reported finding evidence that Maureen had recently been throwing up in the guest bathroom and wondered how he could help her. Maureen was initially tearful and angry that her parents had "snooped" on her. However, she eventually acknowledged that it was true that she was struggling with binge eating and purging again. Her parents were not critical of her and said they understood how difficult it was to stop these behaviors. They asked what more they could do to help. Maureen and her therapist decided to meet independently of Maureen's parents to come up with some suggestions to consider.

A primary aim of the second stage of CBT treatment for bulimia nervosa is to continue to monitor, and to extend if necessary, progress toward, or maintenance of, a regular pattern of eating. The next aim is to help your child delineate the nature of feared and avoided foods and to gradually reintroduce, often with your help, some of these foods into her diet. You can be helpful in these activities by contributing your own observations of your child's behaviors. For example, a feared food—one that is likely to induce binge eating—may be ice cream. You can volunteer to go with your child to get ice cream so that you can be available to support him in eating only one cone and to help him by discussing how he feels about this challenge.

You will probably not be directly involved in the specific activities of problem solving or cognitive restructuring, wherein your child tries to identify strategies to prevent binge eating and purging, as well as problems in her thoughts and beliefs about food and weight. However, you may be a part of some of the solutions that your child and her therapist devise. For example, your child may decide that she has a problem with binge eating when she's alone after school. You may be asked to be available during that time to help prevent binge eating. Or your child's beliefs about attractiveness may overemphasize weight as a focus, in which case you can provide insight and assistance in thinking about these issues in the context of your family.

The final stage of CBT is concerned primarily with the maintenance of improvement following treatment. Progress is reviewed and realistic expectations are established. Relapse-prevention strategies are used to prepare for future setbacks. You can be helpful by identifying upcoming situations that may be stressful and by establishing yourselves as a resource for your adolescent to turn to if things become difficult again. Your involvement in CBT helps to acknowledge the illness and to ultimately reduce shame in your child, so that help (and particularly your help), should it be needed, can be asked for sooner rather than later.

What is your role in IPT for bulimia?

Although adults treated with interpersonal psychotherapy (IPT) are often seen alone, therapists who treat adolescents using this approach would generally include you in the treatment because you play such an important role in the interpersonal dilemmas of your child. Remember that IPT approaches changing disordered eating behaviors related to bulimia nervosa very indirectly. However, IPT is still a very focused treatment, and your importance to the specific tasks is highlighted in the examples that follow.

As is the case with CBT, motivation of the child to attend sessions may be the initial point of entry for parents:

> Sixteen-year-old Felicity eagerly began treatment for bulimia nervosa because she was interested in working on her problems with friends. However, Felicity tended to either forget appointments or show up half an hour late. The therapist discussed how she could improve Felicity's attendance and suggested that her parents could remind her when sessions were scheduled by calling her on her cell phone in advance. Felicity agreed that this would help. Her parents were happy to assist in Felicity's treatment, and this involvement seemed to them and to Felicity to be supportive but not intrusive. In addition, Felicity's therapist had only daytime appointments, and so it was necessary to contact her school (with Felicity's parents' permission) to ask that she be excused from classes for treatment. Contact with the school's counselor helped the school administration to support treatment as well.

In IPT for adolescents there are five main problem areas: grief, role disputes, role transitions, interpersonal deficits, and single-parent families. You are likely to play a role in working on some aspect of each of these areas. The most pertinent for working with adolescents with eating disorders are role disputes, role transitions, and the impact of having only one parent.

Role disputes are differences in opinions about the readiness to take up certain adult roles or behaviors (e.g., dating, jobs). Adolescents frequently act out their role disputes with parents by disruptive, antisocial, or self-punishing behaviors. What differs in helping with conflicts and role disputes with adolescents is the nature of the problem and your involvement as parents. Your child's therapist will attempt to preserve workable family relationships and to provide alternatives to the disruptive

behavior. To do this, it is often useful if you come to some sessions to facilitate the negotiation of these disputes with the therapist present to help you.

Mandy was a 14-year-old who had recently developed bulimia
nervosa. She began to skip school, was caught drinking alcohol, and on two occasions met a male friend late at night in a
park. Her parents were furious at her behaviors and confused by them, as Mandy had previously been a straight-A
student and model child. The therapist helped the parents
and Mandy to realize that Mandy was struggling to assert
herself and develop a sense of independence from her
mother, in particular, who tended to be controlling and
intrusive (mostly out of love and interest). Nonetheless, both
the therapist and Mandy's parents were worried about the
seriousness of the risks that Mandy was taking. Mandy's parents were considering sending her to a residential treatment
setting, where someone "could keep a better eye on her."
Mandy had a good relationship with her therapist and
trusted him to help her. She admitted that she was worried
about her behaviors too at times and didn't really understand why she did such things. She reported that she enjoyed
drinking because it took her mind off her problems but that
she felt vulnerable and a bit stupid for going out late at night
to a park where she might be harmed. Her therapist discussed with Mandy what was happening with her parents
and wondered with her if she was deliberately using these
behaviors to "fight" with them. Mandy agreed that she was
angry at her parents, particularly her mother, who still made
her lunch and bought her clothes for her. She couldn't quite
see how this made her do the things she was doing, but she
did know that her relationship with her parents was stressful
to her.

When the therapist invited Mandy's parents to a session,
the aim was to help Mandy describe how her relationship
with her parents was stressful to her and to help them
to think about how things might change. The therapist
explained that the conflict they were having among themselves was increasing Mandy's discomfort and that she herself recognized problems with what she was doing. During

the session the therapist promoted further discussion of Mandy's anger at her mother, and Mandy was able to express the wish that she be given more age-appropriate freedoms. Her mother agreed to try this, though it would be difficult for her, if Mandy also promised to refrain from drinking and sneaking out at night. This initial session was followed by several others specifically examining the changes the parents and Mandy were making and the effects of those changes on their relationships with one another. Over the next few months, disputes and conflicts diminished and Mandy was more responsible in terms of her risk-taking behaviors.

Both adolescents and adults experience role transitions. Normal role transitions for adolescents include passage into puberty, shift from group to dyadic relationships, initiation of sexual desires and relationships, separation from parents and family, work, college, and career planning. The strategies for addressing role transitions in adolescents do not differ significantly from those used with adults, but therapists will often want and need you, the adolescent's parents, to be included in treatment sessions. The therapist would particularly include you to support the adolescent's giving up a role and to help the family adjust to normative role transitions.

Eighteen-year-old Sally was preparing to leave for college when she was discovered by her mother to have bulimia. Sally's parents were anxious for her safety while she was in college and told her that their payment of tuition was dependent on her seeking treatment. The therapist helped to focus Sally and her family on the importance of the impending role transition that would occur when she went to college. This required that the parents attend several sessions, but the major focus was on the guilt about leaving home and the anxiety about going to college that Sally suffered. To address these issues, the therapist had to help the family acknowledge to one another that this was a significant shift in their relationships and that this change entailed a loss, in the sense that the previous relationship based on cohabitation and day-to-day meetings would be forgone. They were also asked to focus on the opportunity to forge a new relationship with one another based on a more adult way of being together. The parents said that they were worried about how Sally would do without them. They had questions for her about how she would manage the temptations of drug and alcohol use, boyfriends, and commitment to study. Sally, on her part, was patient with her parents about their questions and reminded them that she had some experience with all of these issues and that she had thus far managed them well. She admitted to feeling worry as well, though, about what it would be like to be alone more. Sally's parents described their own experiences of going off to college and were supportive.

Single-parent families (whether resulting from divorce, death, or parental choice) are an added interpersonal focus for adolescent IPT. Not only is the child's relationship with the absent parent affected, but also her relationship with the remaining parent. Interpersonal tasks associated with this problem area include (1) acknowledging that having a single-parent family is a problem to the adolescent, (2) addressing any feelings of loss, rejection, abandonment, and/or punishment, (3) clarifying expectations for how to relate to the absent parent, (4) negotiating a working relationship with the remaining parent, (5) establishing a relationship with the removed parent if possible, and (6) accepting the permanence of the situation.

Fifteen-year-old Monica developed bulimia nervosa approximately 2 years ago when her father gained sole custody of her. Her mother suffered from a substance abuse disorder. Monica had not lived with her father since she was 5 years old. She says her bulimia symptoms have worsened since living with him. The therapist working with Monica helped her assess the importance of her life with her single father as it related to (1) her guilty feelings about having been abandoned by her mother, (2) her anger at her father for not being in her life previously and for failing to protect her from her mother's behaviors while she (her mother) was intoxicated, (3) her wish for a female figure with whom she could discuss her romantic relationships, and (4) her wish to reconcile her parents so they would both be available to her.

As we've said, the treatments discussed in this chapter are focused on helping your adolescent make changes in his or her own behavior while you take a supporting role. In many cases the targeted behaviors are not the eating-related behaviors that are causing your child's health to deteriorate. This means that you should plan on being vigilant in monitoring your child's progress, as well as supportive of the efforts made in therapy. If a child with anorexia continues to lose weight, or one with bulimia continues to binge eat and purge—and especially if these behaviors worsen—you need to take action to get your child medical help quickly and put into effect the backup plan recommended at the beginning of this chapter.

Only time will produce additional data to reveal which types of therapy are most effective in saving lives being damaged by eating disorders. For now, remember that you have a right and a responsibility to be involved in your child's care. In the next two chapters we turn to possible impediments to your being successful in finding ways to help your child, particularly if you are taking direct charge of changing behaviors. The next chapter focuses on working together as parents and the dilemmas with seeing eye to eye on treatment choices and the management of eating-related behaviors. However, even when you overcome your own disagreements as parents, you may find problems in working with your treatment team. So in our final chapter we turn to the difficulties you may face in working with professionals and with staying empowered and effective as parents fighting against your child's eating disorder.

FOR MORE INFORMATION

Agras, W. S., and R. F. Apple, *Overcoming Eating Disorders: A Cognitive-Behavioral Treatment for Bulimia Nervosa and Binge Eating Disorder. Therapist Guide,* 1997. San Antonio, TX: Psychological Corporation.

Fairburn, C. G., A Cognitive Behavioural Approach to the Treatment of Bulimia. *Psychological Medicine*, 1981, *11*(4), 707–711.

Fairburn, C. G., Interpersonal Psychotherapy for Bulimia Nervosa, in D. M. Garner and P. E. Garfinkel, Editors, *Handbook of Treatment for Eating Disorders*, Second Edition, 1997, New York: Guilford Press, pp. 278–294.

Lock, J., Treating Adolescents with Eating Disorders in the Family Context: Empirical and Theoretical Considerations. *Child and Adolescent Psychiatric Clinics of North America*, 2002, *11*, 331–342.

Mufson, L., K. P. Dorta, D. Moreau, and M. M. Weissman, *Interpersonal Psychotherapy for Depressed Adolescents*, Second Edition, 2004, New York: Guilford Press.

Robin, A. L., P. T. Siegel, A. W. Moye, M. Gilroy, A. B. Dennis, and A. Sikand, A Controlled Comparison of Family versus Individual Therapy for Adolescents with Anorexia Nervosa. *Journal of the American Academy of Child and Adolescent Psychiatry*, 1999, *38*(12), 1482–1489.

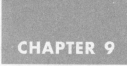

CHAPTER 9

HARNESSING THE POWER OF UNITY

How to Stay on the Same Page
in Your Fight against Eating Disorders

One reason that a good specialist inpatient unit often succeeds in helping children eat normally and, in the case of anorexia, gain weight is that there's a nursing team on hand 24 hours a day to tackle the problem consistently and persistently. This is what you need to do if you're to succeed in helping your child conquer anorexia or bulimia: Unite as a family and stay on the same page, all the time. As we've said before, the fact that children tend to relapse after hospitalization underscores the inability of many families to present the same united front. And with outpatient care being the dominant form of treatment today, it's plainly obvious that parents (with backup from siblings wherever possible) need to learn to come to agreement on exactly how they will participate in their child's fight for health and how they'll stick with it for as long as it takes.

If your daughter is anorexic, you have to figure out how you can develop a united front in getting her to eat. If your son is bulimic, you need to find a consistent path toward helping him eat normal amounts of food and not purge. In Chapters 7 and 8 we showed you what your role might involve if your therapist is using a family approach or another type of treatment to help your child. But even if you adhere to our principles and guidelines, you'll be surprised by how quickly any positive achievements will crumble if you don't spend as much effort on building a united front.

Developing a united front may seem straightforward. You may even feel you don't need this chapter. After all, you know that you and your child's other parent are already in agreement on wanting your son or daughter to get better. Unfortunately, where there's a will, there's not necessarily a way, unless it's exactly the same way and it's well thought out in advance. Wanting to see your child get better is not the same as both of you doing exactly the same thing to make that recovery happen. You and your child's other parent have to "be on the same page" regarding the urgency of the problem, when and how to pursue professional help, what to do at home—deciding what to say to your child to get him or her to eat or to avoid purging, how much food is appropriate, what consequences should be established for lack of progress, how the other kids in the family should be involved, what family sacrifices will be made to facilitate change for the child, and even details such as whether the child has to drink whole milk or skim milk. And you have to stay on that same page every minute of every day.

If you're a typical couple, you may find the idea of being in such constant agreement laughably unrealistic. Most couples have disagreements, some more than others. That's not the issue here. Despite these everyday conflicts, most parents are 100% in agreement that they want their child to recover. The issue here is to figure out how you can work together so that there is no room for the anorexia or bulimia to slip through, as evidenced in many of our illustrations in Chapter 7. Only then will your efforts at helping your child really bear fruit. So, resolve to set your other disagreements aside; on this life-and-death matter, you can agree to agree.

DIVIDE AND CONQUER:
HOW EATING DISORDERS SLIP THROUGH

If it's still hard for you to picture your child's eating disorder slipping through your defenses when both parents are so committed to the recovery process, imagine a fishing net. If the holes in the net are too big, the fish will just slip through. Your family, too, must be tightly woven if you're to keep your child's eating disorder from slipping through. In fact, just like a fisherman, you'll need to check the integrity of your net regularly. Holes have a way of appearing where you least expect them. For instance, you may think you and your child's other parent are saying the same thing while your teenager with an eating disorder hears two different messages.

> Samantha's mother, Jill, says in a strident voice, "For goodness' sake, Samantha, eat now!" Her father, John, rebuffs his spouse by saying, "Don't be so hard on Samantha" before turning to Samantha and saying, "Come on, Sammy dear, just one more bite." Jill and John believe they're on the same page—they've both told Samantha to eat. But clearly the messages are different on the receiving end. Samantha's mother is issuing a command and already sounds angry. John is making a request and treating his daughter with kid gloves, in addition to criticizing his wife.

In cases like this one, which are quite common, the parents are more successful at battling each other than at finding a common strategy to battle their daughter's eating disorder. While Mom and Dad are quibbling about how to get Samantha to eat more, Samantha doesn't have to eat, and the eating disorder is given time to catch its breath, so to speak, or to "slip through." The best way for these parents to get Samantha to eat the amount they want her to eat is for them to really get on the same page. In fact, not just on *the same page*, but *the same line, the same word,* and *the same letter*. This will enable them to speak with one voice and say exactly the same thing: "We know it's hard for you, but we want you to eat more, and we have no choice but to find a way to help you beat this eating disorder."

In the following pages we illustrate a variety of typical disagreements between parents and how you can head them off. We hope that being aware of the insidious ways in which your child's eating disorder will try to divide and conquer the two of you will help you avoid as many of them as possible and quickly resolve those you can't. These examples will also remind you, as parents, to continue to work together in forging a path toward productive efforts to help your child.

If your child has only one parent, you can still gain insight from these scenarios. As we've already shown, you may be getting help from another adult—the child's grandparent or another relative, a partner who lives with you, or even a close family friend—and that person also needs to stay on the same page as you. But even if you're going it alone, you may experience ambivalence over many of the same issues, as Tammy's mother did (see Chapter 7) when she was trying to keep her daughter from purging. Her internal conflict over how much she should control her daughter gave bulimia the loophole it needed to slip through and emerge victorious in the fight for this teenager's health. So, in the following pages, when we refer to your spouse or your child's other parent, we mean to include any other adult who is helping you in this effort.

TYPICAL DIVIDE-AND-CONQUER SCENARIOS AND HOW TO AVOID THEM

1. Only one of the child's parents is convinced that this is the time for action and that they ought to be involved in treatment.

Even though everyone in the family showed up for the evaluation, Mom and Dad argued in the office about whether they should be there. "I'm not sure we should do this right now," Mom said, turning to her daughter, soliciting her agreement. Dad, fuming, said, "I'm tired of pretending that nothing's wrong. When do you think it will be time for us to do something about Rachel's not eating?"

As we've stated several times, most patients do well when their illness has been recognized relatively early on and when both parents realize the need for them to become active participants in their child's recovery. Unfortunately, several factors often work against this potential scenario. Many parents end up immobilized because they feel they are blamed for having caused their daughter's illness. They may feel guilty and therefore think their involvement will only make things worse, or their adolescent is pleading with them not to take her for treatment because she can "handle it" on her own. In that case it's not uncommon for one parent to give in to the pleading of his or her daughter, to express discomfort with "pushing" her into treatment when she so clearly doesn't want to go, or to try to convince his or her spouse that the adolescent isn't ready yet—"she doesn't want to change." The eating disorder is quite good at spotting this kind of opportunity, where rallying the ambivalent parent is often enough to delay any meaningful action, while the adolescent continues to starve herself and the grip of the eating disorder becomes firmer.

This scenario is even more likely to take shape when the adolescent has bulimia. With anorexia, parents can see that their anorexic child looks so obviously unwell. In the case of bulimia, however, it's quite likely that parents will not be aware or will only suspect that food is disappearing or that frequent bathroom trips after mealtimes have nothing to do with "freshening up" but more with their child making herself sick to continue managing her anxiety about weight gain. All these different possibilities, unfortunately, result in the same situation—the parents feel immobilized for one reason or another, the eating disorder is good at taking advantage of this gap, and the adolescent goes without helpful treatment.

If this is the case in your family, what should you do? Try to keep your adolescent out of discussions concerning her health care as much as possible! This may seem unfair to you—after all, she's 16 and you've included her in almost all recent decisions involving her. Unfortunately, anorexia, as well as bulimia to a lesser degree, doesn't allow your teen to think rationally about her need for treatment. Inform your child of your decision, but refrain from seeking her opinion about health care measures. That is what you and your spouse should be talking about. When you two have a private moment, try to sit down to discuss the pros and cons of your child's remaining untreated. It's important to be in agreement, even if this means deciding to "give it another 10 days, but at the end of that time, we will do X, Y or Z," as opposed to continuing to disagree while your child languishes with an eating disorder.

2. One parent's denial is actively colluding with the adolescent's illness.

> Debra's parents have been told that there is little doubt that the diagnosis is anorexia. Dad almost seemed relieved: "I knew it. I was always convinced that this was the problem. We had her visit so many doctors, from the endo guys to the GI docs and back. They couldn't find a thing wrong." Mom was less comfortable with the news: "I think we should go back to Dr. A in the GI clinic. I'm not convinced her regurgitating her food is in her head; there must be something wrong with her intestinal tract. It has to be something with her stomach or such."

Realizing that their child is seriously ill is devastating for almost all parents, so a certain amount of denial is understandable. Some parents, however, find that a diagnosis of an eating disorder remains too uncomfortable to deal with even after they finally come to terms with the fact that their child is unwell. This discomfort often results from the fact that anorexia and bulimia are psychiatric diagnoses. Unfortunately, we still live in a society in which a psychiatric illness carries a certain stigma for some, and perhaps one or both parents will find the thought of their son or daughter's being mentally ill intolerable. In that case it's understandable that parents might prefer to settle for a more acceptable diagnosis such as a gastrointestinal or endocrine disorder or another medical condition. An accurate diagnosis, however, usually leads to the right treatment, which in turn provides the best opportunity for a favorable outcome. It therefore becomes a real treatment dilemma when one or both parents are unable to accept the diagnosis of an eating disorder for their adolescent.

Just as worrisome is that this scenario provides the adolescent's eating disorder with the ideal opportunity to thrive. Earlier in this book we characterized anorexia as ego-syntonic, meaning that the sufferer will often be unable to appreciate the severity of the disorder. In fact, we've known many patients who don't think they are ill at all! Having a parent question the validity of the eating disorder diagnosis only feeds that delusion. In the case of bulimia, the sufferer knows that binge eating and purging are abnormal but is ashamed of the behavior and often tries to hide it. A parent's denial that a problem exists, which often happens, may only make it easier for the child to keep the problem under cover. In both cases, the family is left with a stalemate. With Mom and Dad sitting in opposite camps, the illness remains untreated (or the child is treated for the side effects of her eating disorder rather than the eating disorder itself), perhaps with precious time being lost while the child is dragged from one medical test to the next in futile pursuit of some nonexistent gastrointestinal ailment.

Once again, the crucial issue here is for Mom and Dad to look at the facts together and try to reach an understanding of what the next step in treatment should be. That may be difficult, though, if the adolescent is closely aligned with one parent in such a way that this alliance opposes or excludes the other parent, as is often the case when this scenario develops. The adolescent is "recruited" as an active "consultant" to at least one of the parents, leaving the other parent on the outside and quite frustrated as a result.

Debra's parents need to consult one another, not their adolescent, on these particular health concerns. If you and your child's other parent find yourself mired in disagreement about what's wrong, your child's therapist should be able to help. It's not unusual for us to devote an entire therapy session to getting a parent in denial to see the light.

3. Each parent thinks the other one is not doing enough or doing the right thing to make sure the eating disorder is addressed.

Becky is not gaining weight. Her parents are beside themselves with worry. Instead of focusing on how they can succeed at helping her next time, Dad starts in on Mom, "I told you to give her whole milk. Why do you keep insisting on skim?" Mom then feels humiliated and lashes out at Dad to remind him that he isn't doing "his job": "I asked you to have Becky eat three pancakes at breakfast, but you always seem too busy to wait around till she's done. That's no good either!"

Here the parents have indeed taken action to get their adolescent into treatment and to encourage him or her to eat more. These parents are also heeding the clinician's call that they work as a united team to be most effective in helping to combat their child's eating disorder. However, many couples have disagreements about a variety of issues, including how they should raise their children. So, instead of just being on the same page about how they will manage their daughter's illness, these parents are trying to outdo each other. Helping their son or daughter becomes yet another way in which they battle each other instead of battling the illness. Most adolescents with an eating disorder are quite astute at realizing that Mom and Dad are not quite on the same page, even though on the surface it might appear that way. These parents are making it relatively easy for their adolescent to criticize one parent—"You give me all these foods that you know I don't like"—just to have the other parent join the adolescent in criticizing that parent for not trying harder or being more creative in finding different foods that he or she will eat. Needless to say, the eating disorder's strategy to divide and conquer works well in this family. Next time the adolescent criticizes the other parent, the remaining parent joins in the criticism, and so the cycle continues.

If you find that this happens in your family, you and your spouse should remind yourselves that disagreeing in this way is not going to help your child recover from anorexia. Although you're both trying to get him or her to eat more (which is good and will help him or her gain those much needed pounds), you won't be nearly as successful as you could be unless you can remind yourself that on the issue of how much food, when, or how, you cannot disagree with your spouse at all! Try not to disagree in front of your child. When your spouse says something about food type or amount in front of your child and you don't agree, go along with your spouse for the moment. When the two of you have some private time, discuss your differences frankly and make sure you come to an agreement about how to handle the situation when it comes up again. Always agree in front of your child!

4. One parent blames the other for being too critical of the child with an eating disorder.

> Susan didn't gain weight this week. Her mother seems really upset and says, "I wish you'd tried harder. I just knew yesterday that there's no way you were going to be 'up' at weigh-in today, I just knew it." Susan looks distraught, and Dad quickly jumps to her rescue: "I wish you wouldn't always focus on the negative. You know this isn't easy for Susan!"

In some families, there is tremendous acrimony between the parents, which is a reflection of the nature of their relationship well before the onset of the eating disorder. This does not mean that these parents will not be able to help their adolescent. But their challenge will be to find a way to agree to disagree on many other issues and work out how they are to battle their child's eating disorder as a united team. It's very easy, however, for the adolescent to use these circumstances of acrimony between parents to "protect" the eating disorder. If one can accuse one's parent of being horrible, bad, unreasonable, too strict, or critical, it may be easy to get the other parent to take sides by accusing the spouse of never seeing progress, of always expecting the worst, and so on. The end result is that although both parents want their adolescent to get healthy again, they constantly get caught up in three-way struggles.

If you find yourself in this dilemma, you'll have to put your marital issues aside until your teenager is well again. We realize this is easier said than done. Some parents in these circumstances continually remind themselves that arguments between child and parent often lead to arguments between the parents, and that's how they remain vigilant to the eating disorder trying to slip through. But if marital discord continues to get in the way of your helping with your child's eating disorder, you should consider asking the therapist to help you address some of the crucial issues that make it so hard for you two to agree.

Although it seems fairly typical for one parent to "spoil" a child more than the other, in part because of differences in parenting style (one's permissive, one's not) and maybe also because of favoritism toward one child over the others in the family, you should attempt to find a way to avoid getting into whose approach is right. Instead, agree, as a general rule, that you'll hash out the acceptable responses to your child's food refusal—what tone of voice is appropriate, what words are OK and which are not, how you will remind each other, without being accusatory, when one of you goes beyond those parameters. As we said earlier, you should at least agree not to criticize each other at all in front of your child, but talk about these things only afterward, when alone. The best way to demonstrate your united front is for one parent to say, "Susan, I want you to eat this plate of pasta," and the other parent to immediately respond with, "Susan, your mother and I want you to eat this plate of pasta." In other words, parents should repeat each other's instructions and always try to reiterate that the request for further food intake comes from both of them.

5. One parent addresses the eating disorder with relative harshness, whereas the other constantly tries to soften the verbal blows of the first parent.

"Kate, you have to eat that piece of chicken on your plate," Dad says adamantly. "I hate it when you tell me what to do," Kate retorts. Then she turns to her mother and says, "Tell him not to yell at me. You know I don't like chicken. Tell him, Mom, tell him." Kate's mother knows that it's Kate's anorexia that's trying to divert her attention to quarreling with Kate's father so that the anorexia can have its way. So she doesn't "tell him" as her daughter pushes her to do.

Instead, she says, "We both know you don't like chicken, honey. No one's trying to make you eat food you don't like. Maybe you can skip your meat, just this once."

In this variation on the preceding scenario, the child's eating disorder is again trying to gain a foothold by training the parents' attention on each other and away from the illness that's causing their child to waste away. Here, however, the parents seem to be on the same page, because Kate's mother is onto anorexia's tricks. But not quite. Kate's parents may be on the same page, but they're not on the same line, the same word, and the same letter, as they need to be. They may not have gotten engaged in a dispute with each other, but anorexia did win.

Kate's mother doesn't know what else she could have done. Both parents are trying very hard to get Kate to eat more healthy meals. But if Kate's mother insists that Kate eat what's in front of her, she'll have refused to protect her daughter from her father's "bullying" and will be seen as a bully herself. If she gives in to her daughter's wishes, she'll be opposing her husband's efforts at getting their daughter to eat healthier quantities of food. Kate's mother chose to bargain with the eating disorder and let Kate have a compromise meal—in this case, as is typical, a salad with fat-free dressing or no dressing at all. This scenario leaves Kate satisfied, Dad frustrated with his wife *and* daughter, and Mom embattled for trying to please both her husband and *her daughter* (read *the eating disorder*). The winner, of course, is the eating disorder.

When parents disagree about how to help their child, as these two parents have, they should always discuss their differences in private. Acting out these differences in front of the adolescent at mealtimes will only serve to blow more steam into the already invigorated illness. Even though Kate's mother would have felt uncomfortable with how this meal was proceeding, supporting her husband's effort (demand for eating X, Y or Z), would keep them on the same page. Once these parents have a private moment, they should discuss what's just happened at the table and figure out how to deal with it when this scenario presents itself again.

6. After some progress, one parent gets nervous about the child's weight gain and begins to criticize the other parent's efforts.

Janet's mom and dad did a lot of homework together, reading as much as possible about her anorexia, investigating every treatment option, and pursuing the goal of getting their child back on track with remarkable determination. The therapist had few difficulties in convincing them of what needed to be done to make sure that Janet started eating what she needed to gain the 25 pounds she had lost in the preceding 3 months. Things went well from the treatment perspective, and every week the parents would tell their doctor how they had managed, under difficult circumstances, to make decisions together about how much their child should eat. Janet's weight responded likewise and made good progress, with a pound or so gained every week.

However, as her weight started to approach a healthy level, Janet became increasingly uncomfortable and anxious and accused her parents of feeding her too much and making her fat. Although this was not the case, Dad started undermining Mom's efforts at helping Janet eat sufficient amounts of food at regular intervals. "I don't think she needs to eat quite that much anymore," he'd say. It turns out that Dad was also getting anxious about Janet's weight gain. Mother, in an outburst, accused Dad of being afraid that his daughter would, in fact, become overweight: "I always suspected that you wanted her to be thin. I always knew it."

Some parents appear to be able to work well together from the start, and Janet's parents certainly began on the same page. However, Janet's constant pleading, especially with Dad, not to make her eat, eventually convinced him that perhaps they were, in fact, "making her fat." For Janet to reach a healthy weight, Dad needed a great deal of assurance from the therapist that he and his wife were doing the "right thing."

All parents know well what to feed their child when he or she is starving—it's just that the eating disorder trips them up, getting them to doubt themselves. Therefore, the challenge for

Janet's parents, especially her dad, is to remind themselves and
one another that they usually do know best and should follow
their gut instincts, hang in there, and listen to one another when
it comes to their child's health status. If unsure, they should consult with a professional and not allow their child to counsel them
on her health care needs—after all, she is only 12! Janet, on the
other hand, obviously needs her parents' assurance that they are
helping her, that they only want her to be healthy and happy
again. They must repeat this message jointly to her as often as
needed.

What happened in this family is actually quite common. The
adolescent manages to gain weight in the beginning, as parents
have put up a united front in their efforts to help their child
recover. However, in many instances the adolescent "goes along"
in the beginning, only to find him- or herself getting very anxious at reaching a certain point in weight gain, at which point he
or she "slams on the brakes." The parents' challenge is to continue in their efforts even beyond this point. Their task is not
only complicated at this juncture as perhaps they are tired after a
long struggle, but when one parent "agrees" with the adolescent
that "perhaps this is enough weight gain," then the family has a
real challenge at hand. It's not uncommon for one parent to be
quite anxious about the child's weight gain, as is the case for
Janet's father. In situations like this, parents need to check with
one another about their goals for their child. And, as with everything else in recovery, they need to agree on what weight will be
acceptable. You have to discuss such disagreements and not
allow your own possible anxieties about weight gain to get the
better of you.

7. Divorce or other circumstances have created a parental
   triangle that makes staying on the same page
   almost impossible.

Diane and Lou's divorce was not amicable, and the two have
a hard time speaking, much less spending time together with
16-year-old John, who has anorexia. Diane is the custodial

parent, but she works the 7:00–3:00 shift at a hospital an hour's drive away. So her mother, who has her own home about 5 miles away, comes over at 7:30 to make John's breakfast before he goes to school and to see that he eats it. It's not very convenient, but John desperately needs to gain weight, and she's willing to make this sacrifice. John then has lunch on his own at school and goes to his father's house after school, where he has his afternoon snack under Dad's supervision. He then returns home for the evening and has dinner with Mom. This array of adult caregivers involved in John's eating makes coordination of their refeeding effort extremely difficult, and John's progress has been slow. "I'm sorry," his mother has said repeatedly when their therapist expresses concern about this arrangement. "I love my son, and I'm trying to do the best I can. But I have to go to work early, and there is no way I can get time off. We're already understaffed. If I ask for a leave, I'll lose my job permanently. Yes, of course, I'm worried about John, but his dad and grandmother will just have to help out."

Everyone in this family wants to be involved in the care of the teenage boy they love, but getting all three interested parties on the same page is quite a challenge. When such family members don't necessarily talk with one another (as is the case between Mom and her ex-husband) or live in the same home, their refeeding program is vulnerable to failure no matter how well intentioned everyone is. Because there are so many loopholes in this regimen, it's very easy for the eating disorder to find an escape route and slip through. For instance, John can easily convince Grandma that he doesn't have to have "that much" for breakfast, because "Mom already gave me so much to eat for dinner last night." John does not have to have any lunch at school because there is no one to supervise him there. When he goes to his dad's for his afternoon snack, he can announce that he doesn't feel like eating much "since I had tons of food for lunch at school." In keeping with what we have tried to make clear in previous chapters, it's not that John wants to lie to his parents, but, rather, the eating disorder is being given an ideal opportunity to slip through the cracks of this very "porous" system the adults have put in place. This family system is supposed to help John restore his weight to within a normal range for his age and height.

What needs to happen here to remedy the situation? There are many differences that may have brought on the divorce between John's parents, and Mom may have issues with her own mother because of her having to step in to help with child care. If John stands any chance of recovering from his anorexia, these adults will have to find a way to talk with one another, set their personal differences aside, and figure out how they can work together more successfully in John's refeeding. Their therapist should be able to help them work this out.

One possible solution is for each member of this family, after the meal for which he or she is responsible, to report by phone to the next person in line. Grandma calls Dad and leaves a message telling him what John ate and what he said about it; Dad then decides what is an appropriate snack. Dad likewise makes a call, leaving a message for Mom so she can decide how to handle dinner. That way they don't have to talk to each other in person. Moreover, a school counselor, for instance, could be assigned the task of checking up on John discreetly at lunch to see what he's eating and maybe even offer a couple of words of encouragement. In that case, Grandma could call the counselor directly or could leave a message for Mom and Mom could make the call. Then the counselor could report to Dad.

If this schedule does not work out as planned, and all parties cannot put their differences aside, they may have to return to the therapist, who can serve as a mediator to help them communicate about how best to help John. The therapist could, for instance, designate one of the three as the "point person" who is responsible for communicating with the others and keeping track of what John is eating. In John's case, it could be his mom inasmuch as she's the custodial parent and the obvious choice, or it could be the grandmother because she may find it easier to talk to both of the others than it is for them to talk to each other.

8. One parent is very effective while the other feels defeated.

"I feel I have to do everything to help Karen get better. I know her dad agrees with me that she's really sick, but he's given up and doesn't want to fight this illness anymore. I resent that, because I end up being the one who has to make all the milkshakes. I'm the one who sits with Karen until she has finished her meal. I'm the one who gets up early and makes her breakfast. I think she really hates me, and all the while he gets to be the good guy."

Karen's mother understands the predicament her child is in, and she is taking appropriate steps to get their child into treatment. But she can't take much satisfaction in her accomplishments, because Karen's dad is leaving his wife to feel like "bad cop," on top of suffering the exhaustion and resentment of handling all the food preparation and meal monitoring. Mom is, in effect, battling both Karen's illness and her husband, as the illness has been able to obtain "refuge" in Dad's abdication. This is most unfortunate, for in every setup outlined here so far, one issue is the same—while frustration and despair mount in the family, the eating disorder flourishes.

One parent can be successful at refeeding the child or making sure she doesn't binge or purge, as long as this parent is aware of having the emotional support and understanding of the other parent. Some couples, whether because of personality, temperament, or mere logistics, opt to have one parent do the work. However, the important prerequisites are their agreement on the fact that their child has a serious illness and their willingness to support each other, even if this support means only emotional or psychological comfort.

Every family has its own unique set of circumstances that will determine how it responds in the face of a crisis. The important point is that regardless of this set of circumstances, the parents always have to agree on the seriousness of their child's illness and always have to agree to support each other in addressing the problem. Karen's father seems to agree that his daughter has a terrible illness, but his willingness to give up on fighting it may be his way of denying the full urgency of the problem. Or maybe it's just that he really has exhausted his personal resources for fighting the illness. Like overcoming most potentially fatal or chronic illnesses, battling anorexia or bulimia requires quite a bit of stamina on the part of the parents. That is why it's so crucial for parents to be able to put their differences aside and figure out a way to present a united front. It's all too easy for the adolescent with an eating disorder to spot the differences between parents and capitalize on these differences to allow the eating disorder to persevere. If the "hardworking" parent runs out of steam, there won't be another parent to back him or her up.

It is therefore imperative that Karen's parents work out an agreement whereby they can be supportive of one another. Even if Karen's mother ends up doing all the hard work of refeeding, the chances are greater that she'll be able to persevere *if* she feels Dad supports her efforts in spirit if not in body. If he feels he cannot do what his wife is doing, he should verbally support his spouse and make her feel that he is 100% behind her efforts. And he should do so in his daughter's presence so that her eating disorder knows in no uncertain terms that there is no opportunity to slip through. Being "bad cop" on top of doing all the work will leave anyone depleted.

9. Parents take turns in siding with the adolescent (the eating disorder) against the other parent.

When parents take turns in siding with their child, his or her eating disorder has an ally in both parents but not at the same time. When parents are not used to working together, they may, in fact, find it a little awkward when they do agree. This may be because they aren't used to it, or they don't really want to because they are so used to taking opposing viewpoints. When they're confronted with the prospect of figuring out together how to address their child's eating disorder, they have a real dilemma on their hands. Unfortunately, as in every scenario sketched so far, it's the adolescent's eating disorder that comes out on top. Because the parents in this example cannot see eye to eye, they will instinctively oppose each other, even when there has been progress in defeating the eating disorder. How does this look in practice?

> Dad has been quite successful at working out a schedule whereby he or his wife spends time with Linda after every meal, whether it's watching television together, reading together, or making sure she doesn't throw up the meal she just had. Dad feels quite pleased that he has been able to help Linda not throw up every time he's spent time with her after a meal, perhaps even to Linda's relief. Because of Mom and Dad's long-standing inability to work together, however, even when it might mean helping their adolescent, Mom accuses Dad of being too rigid or too strict with Linda and says, "How can you be supervising her like that? She's not 3 years old." Dad backs off to allow Mom to take the lead in helping Linda. He then finds himself in position to challenge Mom about doing something wrong when it comes to Linda's care: "I think you made her eat that rice too fast," Dad says. "That's why she wanted to purge right after the meal. I think you should give her more time."

In the preceding scenario of endless back-and-forth, Linda's eating disorder doesn't have to do too much to render her parents' efforts relatively futile. This again points to our now familiar argument: It is absolutely essential for parents to find common ground in whatever strategy they feel most comfortable with when they address their adolescent's illness. Think of a well-oiled nursing team in a specialist inpatient unit and how the success of the team members' work is attributed mostly to their ability to speak with one voice and never to second-guess each other when it comes to addressing the eating disorder. If you and your spouse disagree, don't display this in front of your teen. Instead, go along with the spouse who took the first step at normalizing your child's eating. Only later, perhaps after a meal and when you are on your own, let your spouse know that you disagree and discuss a compromise strategy.

STAYING ON THE *RIGHT* PAGE

Sometimes parents are on the same page, but it's the wrong page. They're unified in their efforts and their attitudes, but because they're headed in the wrong direction, the eating disorder is going to emerge victorious.

1. The parents are united, but in fighting their child,
   not the eating disorder.

> "I don't know when to believe John anymore. He tells lies all the time. He says he doesn't vomit, and then I find all the evidence in the bathroom," John's mother says. "Yes, he is really difficult. He's come to be such a negative influence in our family," his dad adds.

We discussed the importance of separating the illness from the adolescent in Chapter 7. For parents to be effective at helping their child through an eating disorder, and for the adolescent to know that his or her parents and the doctors aren't fighting him or her, it's very helpful to see the anorexia or bulimia as something that has overtaken the adolescent. The eating disorder should be perceived as an illness that has taken over his or her life, something he or she hasn't brought on him- or herself, and something that's most certainly not within his or her control. Understanding an eating disorder this way helps parents in their struggle—they are not fighting their adolescent but are battling the illness. So, when your teenager finds a way to hide food, dispose of food, eat an entire cake and not tell the truth about it, or get rid of the food by throwing up, you should remind yourself that he or she isn't a "bad" person and is not willfully trying to deceive you. Rather, his or her illness gets your child to do this because he or she is so dreadfully anxious that weight gain will result if he or she doesn't throw the food away or throw up after a binge.

Naturally, then, when we propose that parents need to put forth a united front, we mean a united front against the illness, not against their adolescent. In the preceding brief example,

John's parents are indeed on the same page, but unfortunately they are united in their disapproval of their son (because *he* lies, *he* hides food, *he* throws up, and so on). In this scenario where the parents do not separate John from his eating disorder, the adolescent is left vulnerable to be overtaken by an illness that controls the way he thinks about himself, his weight, and his shape, and that powerfully influences how he behaves in response to these thoughts. He also has his parents thinking that he's a bad kid for "doing all this." The more these parents fight their child, the more they'll probably feel frustrated and be convinced that "he's doing this to spite us" or keep asking themselves and each other, "Why doesn't he just snap out of it?" The adolescent ends up feeling alone in his predicament and will have a very hard time convincing his parents that he isn't a bad person. All the while, the chances are good that his symptoms will flourish, further heightening the parents' disgust with him for throwing up, for instance, and his despair for being so utterly misunderstood.

These parents' shared inability to separate the illness from their adolescent has made it very difficult for them to be effective at helping their son through this ordeal. John's parents should constantly remind themselves that an eating disorder is no different from any other illness—an adolescent with cancer didn't choose to have the illness, nor is he responsible for feeling miserable, tired, in pain, or for having other illness-related feelings and behaviors.

2. The parents check with the adolescent about important health-related decisions.

Sharon is just not gaining much weight week to week, and her parents can't quite understand why. It turns out that Sharon is very much involved in her own treatment planning. "Yes," her mother explains, "we always ask Sharon whether she's OK with our meal plan." "It's a good thing," Dad adds, "that she has to help us make these decisions because she has to feel she's part of the process. Otherwise, she'll feel left out and won't eat anything."

In commonsense terms, these parents sound as though they're doing the right thing. Their daughter does eventually have to make the right decisions about what to eat on her own, and so it sounds smart to get her involved now. Unfortunately, she's not yet ready. These parents have been checking with their adolescent regarding her views or thoughts on a variety of subjects. Giving your adolescent an opportunity to voice her own views and develop her own ability to make important decisions or choices is part of normal adolescent development. You'd want that to happen for your child, and you've spent many years cultivating a very democratic style of parenting. But when an eating disorder comes along, and *only* in terms of managing the eating disorder, you may temporarily have to take back control, at least until your child is ready to be independent in her eating patterns again.

If your child is not yet an adolescent, habitually involving the child in decision making is more a matter of parenting style than of making a natural transition to the child's evolving independence. In this case you may temporarily have to alter your parenting style. How you will manage your child's eating disorder by changing your parenting style will be a personal decision and will depend on the unique circumstances in each family.

Sharon's parents know that Sharon should have ice cream for dessert. After all, she is terribly underweight, she had very little of her dinner, and she needs more calories to stave off further weight loss. They both know that and agree with one another about the course of action. Still, they can't resist asking Sharon whether she wants the ice cream. This is, after all, a reasonable thing to ask any healthy adolescent, and accepting her answer if she declined would be reasonable as well.

What Sharon's parents are forgetting is that when they talk to Sharon about food, they are not talking to a daughter who has reached the level of maturity expected of a typical 15-year-old, but to anorexia nervosa. And anorexia nervosa will always answer "no." Sharon may very well want the ice cream, but when someone is overtaken by the symptoms of anorexia, she will certainly refuse it—"It's bad for me, it'll make me fat" or "You know I don't like ice cream" are typical responses. The result is that the parents find themselves in an awkward dilemma. They may feel that the alternative to continuing to ask such questions of their daughter is to be unacceptably "mean" or disrespectful of the kind of person she has proven herself to be. "We always let her have what she wants," said Sharon's mother. "She's such a careful and thoughtful child, and we know she'll make the right decision." This may indeed be true for every aspect other than eating, and it may have been true for all aspects of Sharon's adolescence before the eating disorder overtook her thoughts and feelings about food, weight, and shape. But it's not true now, because Sharon is not the one making the decisions about food.

What should Sharon's parents do? They have to *temporarily* find a way to avoid giving Sharon much of a choice when it comes to the foods she eats. If they feel that contradicts their parenting style and they feel they *have* to introduce choices, these choices should be between chocolate and strawberry ice cream, as opposed to ice cream or no ice cream. Although our proposal may seem somewhat dogmatic, chances for the recovery of your adolescent are accelerated when her weight goes up, when she manages to refrain from binge eating or purging her food, and when getting stuck in an endless "eating disorder debate" is avoided.

CAN PARENTS AGREE? THEY MUST.

We've presented several typical disagreements in parents' approach to anorexia and bulimia nervosa, each time pointing out how these disagreements can hamper your child's recovery and how your child might try to steer you away from ultimately helping her with her eating dilemma, by dividing your efforts or by simply distracting you from the task at hand—her recovery. In each example, we've also pointed out what to look for in your own behavior that may, in fact, complicate the steps you've already taken to help your child. Finally, we've shown specifically how you, as parents, can work together in a way that's productive for your child, even if you and your spouse have to agree to disagree for now. We hope you'll use these examples as inspiration in your efforts to find a way to agree on how to help your child, from meal to meal, from minute to minute.

FOR MORE INFORMATION

le Grange, D., Family Therapy for Adolescent Anorexia Nervosa. *Journal of Clinical Psychology*, 1999, 5, 727–740.

Lock, J., D. le Grange, W. S. Agras, and C. Dare, *Treatment Manual for Anorexia Nervosa: A Family-Based Approach*, 2001. New York: Guilford Press.

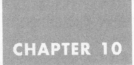

CHAPTER 10

STAYING EMPOWERED AND INFORMED

How to Work with Professionals
Who Are Trying to Help Your Child

Professionals who are trying to help your child will always have your child's best interest at heart. That does not mean, however, that you'll always find yourself in agreement with the doctors when it comes to their treatment plan for your adolescent. You may have to struggle to see eye to eye with your child's pediatrician, psychologist, psychiatrist, or therapist, because in many cases parents are still viewed more as part of the problem than as a key to the solution. So, as much as we would like to believe that you can become a full member of your child's treatment team just by being willing and able to participate, that's not yet the case in all treatment settings. Fortunately, the mindset that resists parental involvement in the care of teenagers with eating disorders is shifting as research data supporting the importance of parents' contribution continue to accumulate. Just be aware that you may have to make a greater effort to stay informed and empowered than you might expect, which is why we've devoted a chapter to suggestions for handling the dilemmas you may encounter during your child's diagnosis and treatment.

Throughout this book we've emphasized the critical need to *stay on the same page* during your child's treatment. In Chapter 9 we looked at what that demands of two parents or other adults raising a child who has an eating disorder. But the concept applies equally to everyone involved and in contact with your child while she is recovering from anorexia or bulimia. Not only must you and your child's other parent be on the same page, so should the members of the treatment team be in full agreement with one another, and with you and your child's other parent. Obviously, this condition can't be met unless you feel your treatment team is on the right course. The value of this *agreement* among all parties should not be underestimated—it is all too easy for the adults (you and the professionals) to become confused about the right course of action to pursue, while your child's treatment suffers as a result. In the last chapter we talked about how the eating disorder can exploit disagreements to derail the efforts to get your child back to health. Anorexia or bulimia can also easily find cracks in the front established by the *entire* alliance formed to help your child—both parents and all the professionals involved. In the next several pages, we detail some potential pitfalls that might make it difficult for you to agree with your child's treatment team, as well as what you can do about such a situation so that you can remain a vital part of the solution. Although it is not possible to advise you on the specific makeup of the treatment facilities or treatment teams in your area, we hope you will read this chapter in conjunction with the information provided in the Resources section that follows and that this can help you to come up with a strategy that will support your efforts to help your adolescent. Finding the best treatment facility for your child will be a challenge, but we hope that having reached this point in this book will equip you with sufficient knowledge to make an informed decision and play a constructive role in your child's recovery.

In addition to the difficulties of parents that are discussed in Chapter 9, the following are common dilemmas that parents encounter, not only in trying to stay on the same page with the practitioners treating their child but also in retaining an active role in the child's recovery. Keep in mind that the central question is not whether the professionals on your child's team are dedicated to helping her get better, but whether their treatment philosophy allows you to be fully involved. If it does not, preparing yourself to stand your ground in a constructive way will go a long way toward enabling you to play an active part in your adolescent's treatment.

A professional you've consulted says your child's problem "cannot be an eating disorder."

There are many reasons that your child's pediatrician or other doctor might make this pronouncement. If you've agonized over the decision to seek help, your child has resisted, and you're sick with worry, this conclusion may initially provide some relief. But relief can quickly turn to increased anxiety when you know that something is wrong and the doctor has left you with no explanation or course of action, especially if, like many parents, you've been doing some research on your own and are pretty well convinced that your child has an eating disorder. What do you do?

To start, consider why the doctor has reached this conclusion. Knowing this can lead you to a next step that will get you on the path to helping your child. Is it likely that this doctor is simply not very psychologically minded and would not ordinarily consider a psychiatric diagnosis? If you have prior experience with the practitioner, what does that history tell you? Has the doctor ever suggested considering psychological factors when your child has had a problem in the past? If not, and he has said something like, "I've examined Rachel very carefully, and I have given this a lot of thought. Although I can't find any medical reason for her weight loss, I just don't think it is an eating disorder," obviously, you'll need to ask him why he doesn't think this is an eating disorder and what you should do now inasmuch as your child continues to resist eating or to binge eat and purge. If the doctor suggests a "wait and see" course, you'll have to make it clear that you've already waited and that you are far too concerned about your daughter's health to allow any more time to pass before taking action. This statement can be firm without being abrasive: "Doctor, I appreciate the care you've taken to consider all the medical causes of Rachel's behavior, but I'm really worried and don't know what to do. Can you refer us to someone who has experience with eating disorders so we can be sure that ruling this out is the right thing to do?"

Another possibility is that despite her best intentions, the pediatrician you have consulted has not based her view on all the available evidence, both medical and psychological/psychiatric. Again, you can ascertain this by asking exactly what the doctor has taken into account—"Doctor, are you satisfied that you've done all the tests to rule out a medical illness that can explain my child's weight loss? We want to be sure that every angle has been considered"—and making your own judgment about how certain the doctor seems and how thorough her assessment appears to have been. Does she respond cryptically, vaguely, or defensively? If so, it may simply be an indication that she is not very comfortable in this area. In most cases, a tactful question along these lines will give the doctor an opening to admit that she's not satisfied with her own finding and will refer you to someone else who can do more.

It's also possible that the doctor has taken into account *only* what the tests and office exam can show—not the behaviors you have observed at home or that have been reported to you by your child's school. Your child's eating habits are not going to be evident in the doctor's office, so what you and others who are around your child much of the day see her doing is critical to a diagnosis of an eating disorder. If you think the doctor has not taken your reports seriously, reiterate them. Many parents benefit from bringing a written log of the behaviors they've observed (what their child has eaten and not eaten at various times during the day, what she has said about food and eating, notable changes in behavior, exercise habits, and so forth) to the doctor's office. If you haven't already done this, and the doctor can assure you that your child is in no imminent danger (see the warning signs on pages 21–22), you might offer to construct such a log for the week ahead and then meet with the doctor again.

Although making a diagnosis of an eating disorder may be straightforward for those who work with these illnesses on a daily basis, many pediatricians and other general practitioners don't have this background. When they've seen very few cases of anorexia or bulimia, they may be somewhat cautious to make this diagnosis. If your child is between 9 and 11 years old, it will be difficult for the doctor to recognize such a disorder even if he or she has been dealing with adolescents with bulimia or anorexia, because eating disorders are quite rare among young children and the manifestation of the illness in them may be atypical. Similarly, eating disorders are not as common among boys or in some ethnic minorities, and again, the pediatrician may not be inclined to consider anorexia or bulimia as a potential diagnosis because your child is male or a member of an ethnic minority.

Unfortunately, diagnoses of eating disorders are overlooked from time to time because it's simply not the first diagnosis that medical professionals will think of—or even consider if they haven't seen anorexia or bulimia before. If your instinct and your knowledge of your child tells you that he or she indeed has anorexia or bulimia, you should ask for a second opinion from someone such as a child and adolescent psychiatrist or a psychologist who specializes in the treatment of eating disorders. You may be hesitant if you feel intimidated by medical professionals, or you fear that your pediatrician will somehow be offended, that you don't trust her. But once you have put your reluctance aside, getting a referral from your child's pediatrician ought to be a relatively straightforward request and procedure. Most doctors would welcome you to explore this option, for they could also learn from the outcome of such an evaluation. If it turns out that a diagnosis of an eating disorder is confirmed, then you should consult your pediatrician about how he or she would like to continue to be involved in your child's medical care. Most pediatricians would want to stay involved in your child's care and would probably be quite happy to consult with your child's psychologist or psychiatrist.

A professional tells you to stay out of, or on the sidelines of, your own child's treatment.

Parents can experience a variety of forms of exclusion, such as not being part of the core assessment and planning phase of the treatment, not being made a part of the solution by meeting with their child's doctor on a regular basis to discuss the progress in treatment, or worse still, being excluded from the treatment altogether. This approach is in stark contrast to most available evidence that supports parental involvement in the treatment of an adolescent with an eating disorder, as we have stated throughout this book. It is, therefore, quite inconceivable that treatment can be successful without the parents' constructive involvement in one form or another. If you need a reminder of the research findings in favor of parental involvement, see Chapter 6.

Many professionals, however, will follow a treatment path that mostly (or only) addresses your adolescent's concerns and worries, while attempting to keep you at bay. Some professionals may even think of many parents as "overinvolved" and "interfering" in the treatment process. It is, therefore, not uncommon to hear parents report that their child's therapist would not meet with them or even (fortunately, more rarely) take their calls. Any of these types of exclusion can be difficult to overcome.

Although there is no "one right way" for parents to be involved in their child's treatment, you should not be excluded from being a part of making these crucial decisions at the outset of treatment. If you are not to be a part of the treatment process, you should still ask the professionals about the balance between addressing the eating disorder symptoms on one hand, and exploring the "underlying issues" on the other. It should be quite acceptable to ask your child's therapist, "Can you explain your reasoning for not including us in the treatment process?" and "Can you let us know how Sandy's medical status will be monitored throughout this process, who will weigh her and how regularly, and how we can be kept informed about her progress, in psychological as well as medical terms?"

Your aim is to make sure that the dire consequences of starvation or binge eating and purging are addressed urgently and consistently. You should be allowed to question the treatment team regarding your child's progress, both in terms of the improvement in eating disorder symptoms and in regard to the role of and emphasis on psychological treatment. If the medical aspects of your child's illness are not addressed, or if you are not informed about the progress in weight gain or cessation in bulimic symptoms, you should insist on being informed in the same way an oncologist would diligently keep parents abreast of how their child's tumor was responding to treatment.

You are given advice you don't agree with.

Regardless of the exact treatment approach, parents often feel uncomfortable about the advice given by the treatment team but don't know whether they can or even have the right to disagree. You may be told that your child's eating disorder can "be treated only in an inpatient setting" or that "the medications we have prescribed are standard for adolescents with anorexia" or that "residential treatment (in another state) is really your only option." You might be surprised to know that many other parents intuitively feel uneasy about such advice but don't think they can second-guess the professional team. "Who am I to question the doctor?" is the reaction that still pops into parents' minds when they don't feel completely comfortable with professional advice; after all, most of us have been brought up to believe that the professionals "know best." Although our advice is not aimed at setting you on a collision course with your child's treatment team, or encouraging you to immediately oppose or question every decision, you should feel comfortable, as a matter of routine, about asking your child's therapist *why* course X as opposed to Y was chosen. You should feel confident in asking your child's doctor why he or she has decided on medication to treat your child's bulimia and why medication A as opposed to B was chosen. Many doctors want to go into detail about their decisions but are prevented from doing so simply because of time constraints. To make sure this doesn't stand in the way of your being fully informed, you can always ask if another appointment, just to talk through all the important issues, would be wise, or you may be able to set up a regular time when you and the doctor can touch base by phone.

Most important, and perhaps more difficult for you to do, you should feel that you can tell the doctor when you disagree with the chosen treatment course. You should, of course, have a good rationale for this approach after you've done your research thoroughly. How you approach this situation is crucial, as you don't want to be seen as antagonistic and you don't want to invite your doctor to react defensively. You may start by saying, "Can you help me understand why you recommend a residential treatment program as opposed to an intensive outpatient regimen?" or "I don't understand the mechanism of the medication you have recommended. Can you explain how this works and why you've chosen this particular path?" With this approach, even though your questioning might be motivated by your disagreement with the doctor's recommendation, you've phrased your disagreement as a question for clarification. This gives your child's doctor an opportunity to provide a satisfactory rationale that may help convince you, or unfortunately, may confirm that you really cannot agree with the chosen treatment path. Most important, you should be prepared to discuss your differences with your child's doctor in an atmosphere of trying *together* to find the best course of care for your child. The likelihood that treatment will be successful is usually enhanced when everyone is in agreement and can enthusiastically endorse the route of care chosen.

Incidentally, when you have doubts about the advice you're being given, be sure to examine your reasons for feeling this way. For all the reasons discussed in Chapter 5 and elsewhere, your adolescent may try to get you to doubt the professionals. Remember, because her thinking and judgment are severely distorted as a result of her eating disorder, she will try to find ways to perpetuate it. So, when the eating disorder speaks for your child, the effort will be to convince you that the doctor who made the diagnosis was wrong and that the treatment team's attempts to curtail the symptoms are ineffective. After all, if you buy into this claim, you might withdraw your teenager from treatment, in which case the eating disorder wins! Treatment is in serious trouble when your adolescent succeeds in getting you to question the treatment and leads you to either seek "alternative" treatment or, worse still, abandon treatment altogether.

You may start out with full faith in your child's treatment team, but the cognitive distortions that mark an eating disorder can make your teenager very persistent in trying to undermine the treatment and the professionals providing it. So, when you find yourself experiencing growing dissatisfaction with your child's treatment, ask yourself whether you have concrete reasons for doubting its effectiveness. If not, and you realize you're being swayed by your child, gently but firmly remind him or her that you, as parents, are in the best position to make treatment decisions, not your child—not just because your child is still under age, but mostly because the eating disorder does not allow him or her to make rational health care decisions. Also, remind your adolescent that everyone (parents and professionals) must be united in fighting the illness and that it's your goal to stay that way to give your child the best possible chance at recovery.

Your adolescent may still feel that you're fighting him or her. In this case, remind yourself to separate the illness from the adolescent: You are battling the *illness*, not your *child*. This thinking will help you stay on course, even when your adolescent puts forward "logical" arguments as to why you should question the interventions prescribed by the professionals.

If, after examining the source of your doubts, you still aren't convinced that the advice you're getting is right, remember that professionals can't always back up their treatment decisions with hard data, especially considering that the research studies on eating disorders are still so sparse, but they should nevertheless attempt to provide you with the reasons behind their decisions. It is *your* child's treatment, and *asking* will make you a part of the treatment effort, and *knowing* enables you to pursue a particular treatment choice with greater conviction. In fact, you might be pleasantly surprised to find that most therapists will be all too happy to take a few extra minutes and have you think with them about the chosen route for treatment.

You've been given conflicting advice.

Because there's no uniform treatment for adolescents with eating disorders, it's relatively common for parents to be told one thing by doctor A at hospital A and another by doctor B at clinic B. Your dilemma, of course, is "What do I do now?" You obviously want to do what's best for your child, but your job is made considerably more difficult with two opposing viewpoints from professionals. If you find yourself in this dilemma, we can only offer some guidelines about finding the right course of action. First, and as we have suggested earlier in this chapter, ask the respective professionals:

- How they've arrived at their particular advice
- Which guidelines they consult as a basis for their decisions
- How many patients they have treated this way
- What the response has been
- Whether this is standard practice among other professionals in this field
- Whether there are published data to support this approach

Although this may seem unnecessary to some, think of the questions you've asked when your child was fitted with her first set of braces; think of the detail the orthodontist went into in explaining "why," "what," and "when." It's quite acceptable to follow the same approach here, even if your child's psychiatrist appears a little reluctant to engage in this kind of discussion. Remember, it's your child's life at stake, and you want to be assured that you are following the right course of action. Second, and again, as we've mentioned earlier, it's important for you to feel comfortable with the advice so that you can endorse the actions necessary to help return your adolescent to a healthy state. This will happen only if the doctor takes some time walking you through the decision-making process. So, trust your gut instinct when you feel this might not be the right treatment for your child, especially in the absence of research or clinical data. *Parents are usually on target!* Pursue your concerns (within reason) until you are satisfied that you can endorse a specific treatment route.

The professionals are not on the same page.

Whereas the preceding dilemma refers to your having made visits to two different clinicians about your child's eating disorder, the difficulty presented here refers to members of your child's treatment team (two professionals under the same roof) not being in sync with one another. We've already mentioned that treatment of an eating disorder is complex, and several professionals should ideally be involved in your child's care (e.g., a pediatrician, a psychiatrist, and a therapist). These doctors could inadvertently confuse you and your child by providing guidance that might subtly differ at times. Possibly the most common issue that arises concerns target weight. Doctor A may say, "She should probably weigh somewhere in the high teens," when your daughter's weight is just over 100 pounds at the time. Another team member (doctor B), in an effort to sound encouraging, may say "We're almost there" in response to the adolescent's begging to know how much more weight she'll have to gain, as she is just over 100 pounds now. Both doctors have the same goal in sight (a healthy weight, given the patient's height and age), but your adolescent will most likely opt to hear from doctor B, "Just 1 or 2 more pounds." You may be confused as well, not quite sure what the "real" message is. Without having to walk on eggshells all the time, doctors who treat patients with eating disorders need to be exquisitely careful about how they phrase information on weight gain issues. Anorexia not only speaks for the adolescent when food issues arise, it also hears for her. So the girl who is told "we're almost there" not only will prefer that message to "we have another 10 pounds to go" because it allows her to delude herself that she doesn't have to gain much more weight, she may also become very upset at the implication. This vague statement of encouragement can set off an alarm—"I must have gained *so* much weight!"—and send her out of the office in tears. It's important that goals be clear and specific and that all the members of the team agree on them.

Unfortunately, you won't be in a position to control much of these kinds of occurrences. However, it's important to understand how the eating disorder gets your child to think and respond to these events and how important it is for you to be able to check with your child's doctor when these misunderstandings arise. Discussing the distress felt by a girl or boy who is very sensitive to any news about weight gain can only further your collective efforts to speak to your child productively. Moreover, understanding this illness can help you to notice when the professionals inadvertently confuse you. Your job is to let the professionals know when this happens.

Although unintentional miscommunication is, unfortunately, a common occurrence, the team members have an obligation to make sure that they "speak with one voice." You, on the other hand, should let your team know when they confuse you about their messages or treatment goals so that ultimately everyone can stay on the same page. This will, we hope, be easy enough. Go back and tell doctors A and B that you're confused, tell them why, and have them clarify the situation. This way, the doctors will be reminded of their oversight and will probably try harder to prevent this from happening again. You should definitely let them know; otherwise, they'll be unaware of the confusion they've caused.

The various professionals involved are not staying in communication when your child has several psychiatric problems requiring multiple treatments.

Treatment of an eating disorder is especially complicated and often involves a couple of professionals at the same time when other psychiatric illnesses coexist with the eating disorder. Having an anxiety disorder or depression in addition to an eating disorder will further complicate your child's treatment. This is a difficult process to manage, whether the professionals who treat your child are all part of the same team at the same institution or are located at different facilities/practices and are collectively involved in your child's treatment. In either case, the treatment team's responsibility is to stay on the same page with one another, even though they represent different professions and may approach treatment from slightly different perspectives. You need to make sure that these professionals all speak to one another *and* to you, the child's parents.

> Fifteen-year-old Darlene loves ballet. She has lost so much weight over the last few months that her pediatrician recommended she not be allowed to dance while her parents are trying to help her gain weight. Darlene is also quite depressed and meets with a psychiatrist on a regular basis. The psychiatrist treats her with antidepressant medication. So far so good. However, the psychiatrist thinks it's a good idea for Darlene to continue to dance because this makes her happy and may also help with her depression. Both of these doctors are obviously trying what they think is best for Darlene. But Darlene has latched onto what the psychiatrist had to say about her dancing, making it very hard for her

parents and her pediatrician to keep her from dancing. These two doctors should have been in touch with one another first, to make sure that they were on the same page before verbalizing their treatment plan to the family.

Although you don't want to be put into the position of having to check on the team to make sure it's doing its job, you want to be reassured that the various professionals involved in your child's care do, in fact, share notes with one another. You will have a clear sign that this is not happening when you hear different directives from two or more members of the treatment team, as in the example of Darlene. If this is the case, you should point out to the person who is ultimately in charge of your child's care that you are confused, as you've been hearing different directives. It's the responsibility of the team leader to clarify such inconsistencies and make sure there is a united front in the battle against your child's illness. Go back to the team leader after a while and check with him or her to see whether the team members have conferred with one another. In that way, you can be reassured that the dilemma has been resolved—at least for now.

Also be aware that there will be times when it is up to you to decide which of two conflicting approaches you feel is best and to steer the entire team in that direction. For example, a medical team may be quite worried about the potential for bone loss and may stress weight gain above normal to ensure that bone loss doesn't occur. The psychiatric team may see this additional weight gain at that particular point as risky because it could lead to an intensified preoccupation with weight and a relapse. You may need to weigh these conflicts for yourselves, to a certain extent, to determine what you believe is the current priority. Similarly, a nutritionist may recommend a particular diet plan, whereas the psychiatric team may see any prescribed "diet" as leading to a preoccupation with food that increases obsessional concerns about eating. It's often up to parents to weigh the pros and cons of these professional options and sometimes force the team in a single direction. When that is the case, you can ask the professional with whom you agree for advice on how to speak tactfully to the disagreeing team member.

Too many cooks in the kitchen?

In Chapter 9 we mentioned that you want, at most, only two cooks in your kitchen (you and your spouse, *not* your adolescent) while you're attempting to normalize your child's eating habits. Likewise, you also don't want too many professionals involved in your child's care. It's incredibly confusing for everyone when a treatment team tries to address every possible angle of the eating disorder at the same time (group therapy, family therapy, individual therapy, medication, refeeding, occupational therapy, exercise therapy). Such a multifaceted approach invariably involves a pediatrician to take care of the medical issues, a psychiatrist for medication management, an individual therapist for psychotherapy, a family therapist to meet with the family, a nutritionist to consult with either you or your child, and so on. There is no research evidence that this catchall strategy will necessarily provide the results you desire. In fact, it can be very confusing and taxing for your child (who may have diminished resources, given his health status), as well as for you. Our advice here is no different from that offered for every scenario described before: You should feel that you can talk to the doctor who is ultimately in charge of your child's care and ask him or her why another professional has been added to the team, what the rationale is for this practitioner's involvement, what the timing of the other practitioner's interventions will be, and what goals the other professional hopes to achieve.

The treatment team tells you they've done everything they could and can't be of further help.

There are very few, if any, circumstances in which a treatment team should give up on an adolescent's treatment for an eating disorder. No doubt, hearing from your doctors that they have "tried everything" will be distressing to you and will put you, as parents, in the awkward position of disagreeing with your treatment team. You will have to try to persuade them not to give up, or you may have to go ahead and look (yet again, perhaps) for a team of professionals who will make another effort to help your child in her struggle.

Remember, the outcome for most adolescents, if they receive good treatment, is positive. The available data show that when properly treated, we can expect most adolescents to recover from their illness. Therefore, you should question the professionals if you're told that "nothing more can be done," "your child is not ready yet," or "she's not motivated to change." Patients with an eating disorder, as a rule, don't want to get better and will not want to work with you and the treatment team in an effort to overcome this illness. Perseverance is of utmost importance if treatment is to be successful. You *and* the professionals must find a way to persist if you want to help your child overcome this illness.

If worse comes to worse, and the team just can't seem to work together, or you have disagreements with the team that you just can't seem to resolve after diligent effort to do so, it may be time to make some changes. How do you know when you've reached that point? If you've truly lost your confidence in the team, and your child is getting worse or making no improvement, it's time to consider a change. Your child's welfare is the reason you're in treatment to begin with, and the effectiveness of treatment should be the priority. Remember, though, that it's hardly ever constructive to suddenly jump from one group of professionals to another, denying any team the chance to make headway with your teenager.

You are sent from pillar to post.

Not every family with an eating-disordered teen lives in a city or state where a multidisciplinary team of specialists is available to help with the child's treatment. Consequently, you may find yourself being sent from one specialist to another, and these professionals are often in another city or even in another state. You may also have been told to have your child admitted to either a residential or inpatient facility hundreds of miles away in another state. Going back and forth like this can be confusing, and you are often left not quite knowing which avenue to pursue or even which of the available options will result in the best outcome for your adolescent.

No doubt, this is a very difficult position for you to be in—

either shopping around your own city or having to think of sending your 14-year-old away to another state. The important issue here is to feel comfortable with the decision that you will be making and confident that you'll be able to stick with the course you have opted for. This sense of comfort won't be possible unless you feel you have done a fair amount of homework regarding the options available and, consequently, that you've made an informed decision. It's critical that you find a facility and group of professionals that have true expertise in treating adolescents with eating disorders. The Resources section of this book can help get you started on finding such a team, but you can also rely on referrals, track records, years of experience, board certifications, and any other criteria you would normally apply to choosing the best possible health care practitioners for any problem your child has.

So, invest in the time to shop around, because when you've made your difficult decision, it's going to be important for you to show the perseverance we just referred to. As we said at the outset of this chapter, this book should help you to be better informed about your child's eating disorder and the treatment options available. When you are in the position of having to shop around or having to send your child away to a treatment facility in another state, you will now feel, with some certainty, that you have taken the best available step.

We've pointed out several times in this book that treatment will probably be most helpful if you're involved in every step of your child's care. Sending your child away to another state for a month or more for the professionals to get his or her weight back on track or normalize his or her eating behaviors may be helpful to your child, but he or she will eventually return home. You will then have to figure out a way to make sure that he or she doesn't relapse. To do so, you need to be involved in the treatment, and you will have to find a way to communicate this to your treatment team. As we said earlier in this chapter, some professionals would like to keep you out of treatment to a large extent. Your challenge will be either to find a team that recognizes the tremendous value parents bring to treatment or to convince a team of the resources you bring that can help ensure that your child gets back on the road toward recovery. Ask the team members how they usually involve families who travel long distances in their treatment approach.

In this chapter we presented several typical challenges that parents of our patients have experienced with professionals who are trying to help their children. These dilemmas have often resulted in the parents feeling confused and disempowered. There is no doubt that such struggles can hamper your child's recovery. In each example, we have pointed out what the source of confusion between you and your child's treatment team might be. In each case, we have encouraged you to find your voice, make sure you remain informed, and remain a part of the solution. We have also pointed out specifically how you, as parents, can work together with your treatment team in a way that will be productive in your child's recovery. In the next section of this book, you'll find resources for getting the best treatment for eating disorders in the United States and other countries.

FOR MORE INFORMATION

Lock, J., D. le Grange, W. S. Agras, and C. Dare, *Treatment Manual for Anorexia Nervosa: A Family-Based Approach*, 2001. New York: Guilford Press.

RESOURCES

The resources provided are not meant to be comprehensive or exhaustive, but should provide guidance in identifying programs and treatment centers in your region. Every effort has been made to ensure that the information we have provided is up to date, but contact information may have changed after publication.

DIAGNOSIS AND TREATMENT
United States

Northeast

NEW YORK

New York State Psychiatric Institute/Eating Disorders Clinic
1051 Riverside Drive, Unit 98
New York, NY 10032
Phone: (212) 543-5739
E-mail: EDRU@pi.cpmc.columbia.edu
Website: www.columbia.edu/~ea12

The Eating Disorders Clinic is part of the New York State Psychiatric Institute at Columbia Presbyterian Medical Center. Offers free treatment to eligible women who suffer from anorexia nervosa or bulimia nervosa and to men and women who suffer from binge-eating disorder. Both inpatient and outpatient facilities. Adolescents welcome for treatment.

Mount Sinai Medical Center
Adolescent Health Center
One Gustave L. Levy Place
New York, NY 10029
Phone: (212) 423-2900
Website: www.mountsinai.org

The Eating Disorders Program provides medical, nutritional, and mental health assessment and treatment for adolescents with anorexia nervosa, bulimia nervosa, female athlete triad, binge-eating disorder, and other types of disordered eating patterns.

Eating Disorders Center (EDC) at Schneider Children's Hospital
410 Lakeville Road, Suite 108
New Hyde Park, NY 11040
Phone: (516/718) 465-3270
Website: www.schneiderchildrenshospital.org/sch_ado_eat_dis.html

Offers treatment for adolescents and young adults with anorexia nervosa and bulimia nervosa. Treatment takes place in inpatient, day hospital, and outpatient settings. The treatment approach is based on the philosophy that effective treatment must address the biopsychosocial needs of the eating-disordered patient.

Unity Health System /Eating Disorders Program
Department of Psychiatry
Mental Health Clinic
835 West Main Street
Rochester, NY 14608
Phone: (585) 368-6550
Website: www.unityhealth.org

This program offers intake assessment, consultation, psychopharmacological evaluation and medication monitoring, case management, and individual and group psychotherapy. Groups will include an eating disorders psychoeducational group, and contemplation, symptom interruption, relational therapy, binge-eating disorder, multifamily, skills training, and women's groups.

Children's Hospital/Eating Disorders Program
Darlene Atkins, PhD, Director
Adolescent Medicine/Eating Disorders Program
Children's Hospital
111 Michigan Avenue NW
Washington, DC 20010
Phone: (202) 884-5544
Website: www.dcchildrens.com/ProgramAndServices/Program_
    EatingDisordersClinic.asp

The Eating Disorders Clinic sees preadolescent and adolescent (ages 10–21 years) patients with suspected eating disorders such as anorexia nervosa, bulimia nervosa, binge-eating disorder, or obesity. Patients are typically evaluated by the multidisciplinary team, consisting of a psychologist, an adolescent medicine physician, and a nutritionist.

PENNSYLVANIA

Renfrew Center Foundation
475 Spring Lane
Philadelphia, PA 19128
Phone: (877) 367-3383
Fax: (215) 482-2695
E-mail: foundation@renfrew.org
Website: www.renfrew.org

The Renfrew Center Foundation is a tax-exempt, nonprofit organization advancing the education, prevention, research, and treatment of eating disorders. Ages 14 and up.

Friends Hospital/Eating Disorders Unit
4641 Roosevelt Boulevard
Philadelphia, PA 19124
Phone: (215) 831-7845

Offers both partial hospital day treatment program and an outpatient program with both group and individual treatment. Support groups include both patients with anorexia and patients with bulimia. Ages 13 and up.

Eating Disorder Treatment Centers
255 South 17th Street
Philadelphia, PA 19103
Phone: (215) 772-3001
Contact: Michael Pertschuk, MD

Provides comprehensive services for eating-disordered patients. Ages 14 and over.

Center for Overcoming Problem Eating (COPE)
Western Psychiatric Institute and Clinic
University of Pittsburgh Medical Center
3811 O'Hara Street
Pittsburgh, PA 15213
Phone: (412) 246-5117

The COPE program provides comprehensive assessments for individuals (including adolescents 18 and under) and treatment designed to address the specific needs of patients requiring different levels of care.

CONNECTICUT

Yale Center for Eating and Weight Disorders
P.O. Box 208205
New Haven, CT 06520-8205
Phone: (203) 432-4610
E-mail: ycewd@yale.edu
Website: www.yale.edu/ycewd

YCEWD serves men and women who experience problems related to food, eating, weight, and body image. Operated by the Yale University Department of Psychology, it provides services to members of the community, trains doctoral students in clinical psychology, and does clinical research to better understand eating and weight disorders. Provides treatment and therapy evaluation as well as information and referral. Mostly adults, but the center does see adolescents ages 16 and up.

Renfrew Center Foundation
436 Danbury Road
Wilton, CT 06897
Phone: (800) RENFREW
Website: www.renfrew.org

The Renfrew Center Foundation is a tax-exempt, nonprofit organization advancing the education, prevention, research, and treatment of eating disorders. Ages 14 and up.

Harvard Medical School Eating Disorders Center
Harvard Eating Disorders Center, WACC 725
15 Parkman Street
Boston, MA 02114
Phone: (617) 236-7766
E-mail: info@hedc.org
Website: www.hedc.org

A national nonprofit organization dedicated to research and education. It seeks to expand knowledge about eating disorders, their detection, treatment, and prevention and to share that knowledge with the community at large. At the heart of the center's program is a commitment to promote the healthy development of children, young women, and all at risk.

Center for Eating Disorders
St. Joseph Medical Center
7601 Osler Drive
Towsen, MD 21204
Phone: (410) 337-1212
Website: www.eating-disorders.com

A range of services are offered.

South

NORTH CAROLINA

Duke University Eating Disorders Program
Box 3842
Duke University Medical Center
Department of Psychiatry
Durham, NC 27710
Phone: (919) 668-7301
E-mail: eatingdisorders@mc.duke.edu
Website: eatingdisorders.mc.duke.edu

The Duke University Eating Disorders Program emphasizes the implementation of empirically validated treatments for anorexia nervosa, bulimia nervosa, and binge-eating disorder. It offers family, individual, and group therapy; a skills-based group program for parents; nutrition services; medical management; and a variety of educational workshops.

University of North Carolina/Chapel Hill Eating Disorders Program
School of Medicine
Department of Psychiatry
University of North Carolina at Chapel Hill
Chapel Hill, NC 27599
Phone: (919) 966-8721
Website: www.med.unc.edu/psych/clinicalservices/
     eatingdisorders.htm

Offers a comprehensive and specialized approach to the treatment of anorexia nervosa, bulimia nervosa, and related conditions for individuals over the age of 14. Provides the most current and state-of-the-art evidence-based treatments to help individuals suffering from eating disorders achieve a lasting recovery, through intensive inpatient, day treatment, and outpatient services.

LOUISIANA

Eating Disorders Treatment Center
River Oaks Hospital
1525 River Oaks Road West
New Orleans, LA 70123
Phone: (800) 366-1740 *or* (504) 734-1740
Fax: (504) 733-7020
Website: www.riveroakshospital.com/eatingdisorder/index.htm

In association with Tulane University, the Eating Disorders Treatment Center provides comprehensive inpatient and partial hospitalization programs for anorexia, bulimia, and related eating disorders, as well as specialized care for males, females, adolescents, and adults.

Midwest

ILLINOIS

Eating Disorders Program at the University of Chicago Hospitals
Department of Psychiatry, MC 3077
University of Chicago
5841 South Maryland Avenue
Chicago, IL 60637
Phone: (773) 834-5677
Website: www.psychiatry.uchicago.edu/clinical/clinics/edp

Provides comprehensive outpatient and limited inpatient services for the assessment, treatment, and follow-up of adolescents and adults with eating disorders.

MISSOURI

Anorexia/Bulimia Treatment and Education Center
621 South New Ballas Road, Suite 7019B
St. Louis, MO 63141
Phone: (314) 569-6898

Free support groups are available at ABTEC, as is evaluation for admission to a hospital psychiatric unit.

McCallum Place on the Park
Eating Disorders Treatment Programs
100 South Brentwood, Suite 350
Clayton, MO 63105
Phone: (314) 863-7700
Fax: (314) 863-7701
Director: Kim McCallum, MD

This program consists of outpatient, day treatment, residential, and subacute care treatments for adolescents and adults with eating disorders and related conditions.

MINNESOTA

Emily Program
Court International Building
2550 University Avenue West, Suite 314N
St. Paul, MN 55114
Phone: (651) 645-5323
Fax: (651) 647-5135
E-mail: info@emilyprogram.com

St. Louis Park Location
1660 South Highway 100, Suite 141
St. Louis Park, MN 55416
Same contact numbers.
Website: www.emilyprogram.com

The Emily Program is an outpatient treatment program that provides comprehensive psychological, nutritional, and medical care for individuals with eating disorders.

Eating Disorders Institute
Methodist Hospital and University of Minnesota
6490 Excelsior Boulevard
St. Louis Park, MN 55426
Phone: (952) 993-6200
Website: www.parknicollet.com

The program consists of inpatient, partial hospitalization, intensive outpatient, and outpatient treatments for eating disorders.

NEBRASKA

Eating Disorder Program
Children's Hospital
Creighton University Medical Center
8200 Dodge Street
Omaha, NE 68114
Director: Mae Sokol, MD
Phone: (402) 955-6190
Fax: (402) 955-6195
Website: www.chomoha.org

The program consists of an inpatient program, partial hospitalization, and outpatient treatments specializing in children and adolescents with eating disorders.

NORTH DAKOTA

University of North Dakota/Eating Disorders Institute
School of Medicine and Health Sciences
University of North Dakota
120 8th Street, South
Fargo, ND 58103
Phone: (701) 234-4111
Website: meritcare.com *or* www.med.und.nodak.edu

The Eating Disorders Institute is a cooperative program between MeritCare, the Neuropsychiatric Research Institute, and the University of North Dakota School of Medicine and the Health Sciences Center. The group evaluates, treats, and conducts research on eating disorders and obesity. Adults and adolescents 12 and up.

OKLAHOMA

Laureate
6655 South Yale
Tulsa, OK 74136
Phone: (800) 322-5173 *or* (918) 298-7804
Website: www.laureate.com

Laureate's program incorporates the twelve-step philosophy with other treatment modalities.

WISCONSIN

Rogers Memorial Hospital
Eating Disorder Services
34700 Valley Road
Oconomowoc, WI 53066
Phone: (800) 767-4411
Fax: (262) 646-3158
Website: www.neoshofasthealth.com/
    goto.php?url=www.rogershospital.org

Provides men and women with comprehensive, effective treatment for
eating disorders. Offers three levels of care—inpatient, residential, and
partial hospitalization—and all follow a multidisciplinary program with
individualized treatment plans. Offers the only residential treatment
with a separate program for males. Also offers outpatient referrals and
an alumni association.

IOWA

Eating and Weight Disorder Program
University of Iowa Hospitals and Clinics
200 Hawkins Drive
Iowa City, IA 52242
Phone: (319) 356-1354
Website: www.uihealthcare.com/depts/med/psychiatry/divisions/
    eatingdisorders

Diagnosis and comprehensive treatment of all eating disorders.

KANSAS

Menninger Clinic
P.O. Box 829
Topeka, KS 66601-0829
Phone: (800) 351-9058 *or* (913) 273-7500, ext. 5311

The Menninger Clinic offers services for individuals (including adolescents) and a structured, 4-week, comprehensive program.

Southwest

TEXAS

University of Texas, Southwestern
Eating Disorders Services
Children's Medical Center
1935 Motor Street, 5th Floor
Dallas, TX 75235
Phone: (214) 456-5900
Website: www8.utsouthwestern.edu/utsw/cda/dept28702/files/
    78274.html

Offers comprehensive diagnostic evaluation and treatment of anorexia nervosa, bulimia, and related disorders. Uses a multidisciplinary treatment approach with an emphasis on intensive outpatient group treatment where possible to minimize the need for more restrictive levels of care.

West

WASHINGTON

Eating Disorders Program
Children's Hospital and Regional Medical Center
Department of Child and Adolescent Psychiatry and Behavioral
    Health
4800 Sand Point Way NE
Seattle, WA 98195
Phone: (206) 987-2760
Website: depts.washington.edu/adolmed/clinics/edclinic.htm

The Children's Hospital Eating Disorders Program is a multidisciplinary program for the comprehensive treatment of anorexia nervosa and bulimia nervosa. The program provides a continuum of care with available inpatient, outpatient, and day treatment services, depending on the level of care needed by an individual.

CALIFORNIA

Center for Discovery and Adolescent Change
The Eating Disorders Program
9844 Pangborn Avenue
Downey, CA 90240
Phone: (562) 622-1083
Fax: (562) 622-1173
E-mail: eatingdisorders@centerfordiscovery.com
Website: www.eatingdisordersprogram.com

This is a comprehensive residential treatment program dedicated solely to the treatment of adolescent eating disorders.

Eating Disorders Program/UCLA
Neuropsychiatric Institute and Hospital
University of California, Los Angeles
760 Westwood Plaza
Los Angeles, CA 90024
Phone: (310) 267-2572 *or* (310) 825-9989
Contact: Michael Strober, MD

Offers comprehensive services to adults and adolescents ages 12–29, using dynamic, expressive, and cognitive-behavioral therapies. Inpatient and outpatient services.

Montecatini
2516 La Costa Avenue
Rancho La Costa, CA 92009
Phone: (760) 436-8930

This is a female-only treatment center for eating disorders and chemical dependency. It has a twelve-step orientation and is group therapy based.

Eating Disorders Clinic/Stanford University School of Medicine
Child and Adolescent Psychiatry Clinic
Department of Psychiatry and Behavioral Sciences
Stanford University School of Medicine
300 Pasteur Drive
Stanford, CA 94305
Phone: (650) 723-4000
Website: www-cap.stanford.edu

Offers thorough diagnostic evaluations as well as treatment plans. Treatment plans are based on current scientific research and reflect the values, needs, and resources of the child and family. They often include the following therapeutic approaches: individual therapy, family therapy, group therapy, behavioral therapy, parent counseling, and medication therapy.

Eating Disorders Program
Summit Psychotherapy Associates
1329 Howe Avenue, #210
Sacramento, CA 95825
Phone: (916) 920-5276
Fax: (916) 920-5221

Intensive outpatient eating disorders program for adults with individual, group, family, and nutritional components.

Canada

Dalhousie University Medical School
Eating Disorders Clinic
Department of Psychiatry
IWK Health Centre Child and Adolescent Mental Health Program
5850 University Avenue
P.O. Box 3070
Halifax, Nova Scotia B3J 3G9, Canada
Phone: (902) 470-8375
Fax: (902) 470-8937
Website: psychiatry.medicine.dal.ca/clinical/iwk.htm

A multidisciplinary team helps its young clients deal with the physical and psychological consequences of anorexia nervosa and bulimia. The team is involved with direct clinical services and consultation and in developing education programs.

Queens University Eating Disorders Clinic
Brock V, Room 546
Hotel Dieu Hospital
166 Brock Street
Kingston, Ontario K7L 5G2, Canada
Phone: (613) 544-3400, ext. 2548
Fax: (613) 547-1501
Website: meds.queensu.ca/medicine/psychiatry/eatdsr.htm

A comprehensive assessment is followed by psychoeducational groups, individual nutrition counseling, family intervention, and, when necessary, admission to the inpatient unit for stabilization. Consultation from pediatrics is available upon request.

Hospital for Sick Children/Eating Disorder Program
555 University Avenue
Toronto, Ontario M5G 1X8, Canada
Contact: Heather Graham
Phone: (416) 813-7195
Website: www.sickkids.on.ca

An interdisciplinary program for the evaluation and treatment of children and adolescents with eating disorders. Evaluates and treats young people ages 17.5 years and younger who have anorexia nervosa, bulimia nervosa, or an unspecified eating disorder. Offers inpatient, outpatient, and consultative services.

Children's Hospital of Eastern Ontario/Eating Disorders Program
401 Smyth Road
Ottawa, Ontario K1H 8L1, Canada
Phone: (613) 738-5890
Website: www.cheo.on.ca

The CHEO Eating Disorders Program requires a doctor's referral and includes outpatient services, day treatment program, inpatient services, and parent support group.

Bellwood Health Services, Inc.
1020 McNicoll Avenue
Toronto, Ontario M1W 2J6, Canada
Phone: (800) 387-6198 *or* (416) 495-0926
E-mail: info@bellwood.ca
Website: www.bellwood.ca

Provides treatment for people with eating disorders and a variety of compulsive or problematic behaviors. Although its premier treatment center is in Toronto, it has helped clients from all provinces across Canada, the United States, and other countries.

Westwind Eating Disorder Centre
458 14th Street
Brandon, Manitoba R7A 4T3, Canada
Phone: (888) 353-3372 (toll free in North America) *or* (204) 728-2499
E-mail westwindedrc@mb.sympatico.ca
Website: www.westwind.mb.ca

Provides counseling and treatment for individuals suffering from anorexia, bulimia, and related disorders in a home-like atmosphere, significantly different from the institutional format of traditional hospitals and clinics. Treatment is collaborative rather than imposed, uses various interactive techniques, and is individualized and personal.

Child and Adolescent Mental Health Care Eating Disorders Program
The University of Western Ontario
London Health Sciences Centre
6 East, Tower 1, Room 6139
800 Commissioners Road East
London, Ontario, N6C 2V5, Canada
Phone: (519) 667-6640

United Kingdom

**Great Ormond Street Hospital for Children NHS Trust/Eating
    Disorders Program**
Department of Psychological Medicine
Great Ormond Street
London WC1N 3JH, United Kingdom
Phone: 7829 8679
Website: www.ich.ucl.ac.uk/clinserv/dcamhs/fed_eds_parents.htm

The eating disorders team at Great Ormond Street Hospital includes
medical and nursing staff, family therapists, psychotherapists, and psychologists. Its approach to treatment is to help the young person reach
a healthy weight and to eat healthily, to correct any medical problems
that may occur as a result of the eating disorder, and to help the young
person talk about his or her feelings and learn healthier ways of coping
with problems.

St. George's Eating Disorders Service
St. George's Hospital
Child and Adolescent Service
Harewood House
Springfield University Hospital
61 Glenburnie Road
Tooting SW17 7DJ, United Kingdom
Phone: 8682 6747
Website: www.careline.org.uk/Doc.asp?WSDOCID=1390

Treatment is provided on an outpatient, day patient, or inpatient basis,
depending on need. Patients will normally be seen within 1 week of
referral, always within 2 weeks, and in emergencies can be seen within
24 hours. This service is suited to all patients under 16 years of age and
to some 16 and 17 years of age.

University of London/Eating Disorders Unit
Kings College, Box 059
The Maudsley Hospital Institute of Psychiatry
De Crespigny Park
London SE5 8AF, United Kingdom
Phone: 7848 0134
E-mail: edu@iop.kcl.ac.uk
Website: www.iop.kcl.ac.uk

The Institute of Psychiatry's Eating Disorders Unit provides a range of high-quality services for patients of all ages and across the spectrum of eating disorders.

Royal Free Hospital
Middlesex University Royal Free Hospital
Pond Street
London NW3 2XA, United Kingdom
Phone: 8411 5898
Website: www.royalfree.nhs.uk

The hospital has a multidisciplinary child and adolescent service. Comprehensive services are provided for the whole range of child and adolescent problems. The service also has an eating disorders team.

Leicester University/The Eating Disorders Service
Division of Psychiatry
University Road
Leicester LE1 7RH, United Kingdom
Phone: 6252 2522
Fax: 6252 2200
Website: www.le.ac.uk

The Eating Disorders Service is one of the few national and international centers of excellence for these conditions. The department supports research into all aspects of eating disorders, including trials of treatment.

St. Mary's Hospital
Praed Street
London W2 1NY, United Kingdom
Dr. Matthew Hodes
Phone: 7723 1081

Guy's Hospital
St. Thomas' Street
London SE1 9RT, United Kingdom
Phone: 7188 7188
Website: www.guysandstthomas.nhs.uk

Australia

University of Monash/Eating Disorders Group
Department of Pediatrics
Child and Adolescent Psychiatry
Level Four, Monash Medical Centre
Clayton Road
Clayton 3168, Australia
Phone: 9594 4497
Fax: 9594 6259

This group will be running all year and is designed as a peer support group.

Wesley Health Services
Wesley Private Hospital
91 Milton Street
Ashfield, NSW 2131, Australia
Phone: 9716 1400
Fax: 9799 6585
Website: www.wesleymission.org.au/centres/wesleyhospital

Carlingford Day Therapy Centre
3 Dalmar Place
Carlington, NSW 2118, Australia
Phone: 9874 4566
Website: www.wesleymission.org.au/centres/carlingford

The Eating Disorders Day Program (EDDP) operates at both Ashfield and Carlingford locations. The program emphasizes the complete restoration of normal weight gain, retraining in normal eating behavior, and ongoing personal and family cognitive therapy. It also offers an inpatient eating disorders program.

Children's Hospital at Westmead
Locked Bag 4001
Westmead 2145, Sydney, New South Wales, Australia
Contact: Dr. Michael Kohn
Phone: 9845 2446
Fax: 9845 2517
E-mail: davidb3@chw.edu.au
Website: www.chw.edu.au

Eating disorder and weight management programs. Services for adolescents up to 16 years old.

EDUCATION/ADVOCACY/REFERRAL
United States

Something Fishy: Website on Eating Disorders
Website: www.somethingfishy.org/#top

This website is dedicated to raising awareness with bulletin boards, online chats and support, information and referral.

Anorexia Nervosa and Related Eating Disorders, Inc.
Website: www.anred.com

ANRED is a nonprofit organization that provides information about anorexia nervosa, bulimia nervosa, binge-eating disorder, and other less well known food and weight disorders. Its material includes self-help tips and information about recovery and prevention.

AABA—American Anorexia/Bulimia Association
165 West 46th Street, #1108
New York, NY 10036
Phone: (212) 575-6200

AABA provides treatment referrals and educational outreach.

Eating Disorders Coalition
611 Pennsylvania Avenue SE, #423
Washington, DC 20003-4303
Phone or fax: (202) 543-9570
Website: www.eatingdisorderscoalition.org

The Eating Disorders Coalition for Research, Policy, and Action is a cooperative of professional and advocacy-based organizations committed to federal advocacy on behalf of people with eating disorders, their families, and professionals working with these populations.

American Academy of Child and Adolescent Psychiatry
3615 Wisconsin Avenue NW
Washington, DC 20016-3007
Phone: (202) 966-7300
Fax: (202) 966-2891
Website: www.aacap.org

The mission of AACAP is to promote mentally healthy children, adolescents, and families through research, training, advocacy, prevention, comprehensive diagnosis and treatment, peer support, and collaboration.

National Institutes of Health (NIH)
9000 Rockville Pike
Bethesda, MD 20892
Phone: (301) 496-4000
Website: www.nih.gov

The National Institutes of Health is the steward of medical and behavioral research in the United States. It is an agency of the U.S. Department of Health and Human Services.

American Anorexia/Bulimia Association of Philadelphia
P.O. Box 1287
Langhorne, PA 19047
24-hour information helpline: (215) 221-1864
Fax: (215) 702-8944
Website: www.aabaphila.org

This nonprofit provides services and programs for anyone interested in or affected by anorexia, bulimia, and/or related disorders. Its purpose is to aid in the education and prevention of these life-threatening disorders. In addition, referral programs and support groups assist in the treatment and recovery process.

Alliance for Eating Disorders Awareness
P.O. Box 13155
North Palm Beach, FL 33408-3155
Phone: (561) 841-0900
Fax: (561) 881-0380
E-mail: info@eatingdisorderinfo.org
Website: www.eatingdisorderinfo.org

Disseminates educational information to parents and caregivers about the warning signs, dangers, and consequences of anorexia, bulimia, and related disorders.

Academy for Eating Disorders
6728 Old McLean Village Drive
McLean, VA 22101
Phone: (703) 556-9222
Fax: (703) 556-8729
Website: aed@degnon.org

An international transdisciplinary professional organization that promotes excellence in research, treatment, and prevention of eating disorders. Provides education, training, and a forum for collaboration and professional dialogue.

National Association of Anorexia Nervosa and Associated Disorders
Box 7
Highland Park, IL 60035
Phone: (847) 831-3438
Fax: (847) 433-4632
E-mail contacts:
Advocacy: anadadvocacy@aol.com
Hotline: anad20@aol.com
Media: media@anad.org
Website: www.altrue.net/site/anadweb

Provides hotline counseling, a national network of free support groups, referrals to health care professionals, and education and prevention programs to promote self-acceptance and healthy lifestyles. All services are free of charge. ANAD also lobbies for state and national health insurance parity and undertakes and encourages research.

Eating Disorder Referral and Information Center
2923 Sandy Pointe, Suite 6
Del Mar, CA 92014-2052
Phone: (858) 792-7463
E-mail: ed@edreferral.com

Provides referrals to eating disorder practitioners, treatment facilities, and support groups. Referrals to eating disorder specialists are offered at no charge as a community service.

National Eating Disorders Association
603 Stewart Street, Suite 803
Seattle, WA 98101
Phone: (206) 382-3587
E-mail: info@NationalEatingDisorders.org
Website: www.nationaleatingdisorders.org

The largest not-for-profit organization in the United States working to prevent eating disorders and provide treatment referrals to those suffering from anorexia, bulimia, and binge-eating disorder and those concerned with body image and weight issues.

Sacramento Eating Disorders Outreach Program
Mercy Women's Center
650 Howe Avenue, Suite 400
Sacramento, CA 95825
Phone: (916) 733-6315
Fax: (916) 921-7569
Website: www.sedop.org
Contact: Jennifer Lombardi, Executive Director

The program is designed to prevent eating disorders through educational initiatives in middle schools, high schools, and colleges.

Society for Adolescent Medicine
1916 Copper Oaks Circle
Blue Springs, MO 64015
Phone: (816) 224-8010
Website: www.adolescenthealth.org

A multidisciplinary organization of professionals committed to improving the physical and psychosocial health and well-being of all adolescents.

Canada

National Eating Disorder Information Centre
CW 1-211, 200 Elizabeth Street
Toronto, Ontario M5G 2C4, Canada
Phone: 866-NEDIC-20 (toll free) *or* (416) 340-4156
Fax: (416) 340-4736
E-mail: nedic@uhn.on.ca
Website: www.nedic.ca

A Toronto-based nonprofit organization that provides information and resources on eating disorders and weight preoccupation.

Eating Disorders Association of London
635 Wellington Street, Upper
London, Ontario N6A 3R8, Canada
Phone: (519) 434-7721
Helpline: (519) 685-8343
E-mail: edal@canada.com
Website: www.eating-disorder.org/edal.html

The resource center provides a library, support groups, a speaker's bureau, educational workshops, outreach, information and referral about treatment centers, therapists, and nutritionists, as well as drop-in support.

ANAB—Anorexia Nervosa and Bulimia Association–Ontario
767 Bayridge Drive
P.O. Box 20058
Kingston, Ontario K7P 1CO, Canada
Phone: (613) 547-3684

ANAB—Anorexia Nervosa and Bulimia Association–Quebec
114 Donegani Boulevard
Pointe Claire, Quebec H9R 2V4, Canada
Phone: (514) 630-0907
Fax: (514) 630-1225

Eating Disorders Association of Manitoba Inc. (EDAM)
P.O. Box 34099 RPO Fort Richmond
Winnipeg, Manitoba R3T 5T5, Canada
Phone: (204) 888-3326
Website: www.edam.mb.ca/welcome_to_edam.htm

EDAM is a provincial nonprofit organization that provides support for individuals who have a loved one who suffers from an eating disorder. Family members, health care providers, educators, and the general public are invited to join as members, attend monthly meetings, and participate in prevention and awareness activities.

Hopewell/The Eating Disorders Support Centre of Ottawa
Heartwood House
153 Chapel Street, Suite 202
Ottawa, Ontario K1N 1H5, Canada
Phone: (613) 241-3428
Fax: (613) 241-0850
E-mail: hopewell@hopewell.on.ca
Website: www.hopewell.on.ca

Provides persons affected by eating disorders with support and resources they need throughout the treatment and recovery process.

United Kingdom

National Centre for Eating Disorders
54 New Road, Esher
Surrey KT10 9NU, United Kingdom
Phone: 1372 469 493
Website: www.eating-disorders.org.uk

An independent organization set up to provide solutions for all eating problems, including binge eating, bulimia, and anorexia. Services include counseling, professional training, and information for students, journalists, and carers.

Eating Disorders Association
First Floor, Wensum House
103 Prince of Wales Road
Norwich NR1 1DW, United Kingdom
Phone: 1603 621 414
Fax: 1603 664 915
E-mail: info@edauk.com

The leading organization providing information, help, and support across the United Kingdom, for people whose lives are affected by eating disorders. Aims to positively influence public understanding and policy.

Somerset and Wessex Eating Disorders Association
Strode House, 10 Leigh Road
Street, Somerset BA16 0HA, United Kingdom
Phone: 1458 448 600
Website: www.swedauk.org/index.htm

Provides resources and informal, nonstigmatizing services that reflect the needs of the community. Offers a telephone helpline, drop-in, community support workers, and library services.

European Council on Eating Disorders
Department of General Psychiatry
St. George's Hospital Medical School
London SW17 ORE, United Kingdom
Phone: 8725 5528
Fax: 8725 3350
E-mail: eced@sghms.ac.uk
Website: www.eced.org.uk

Formed in 1989 out of a desire for more dialogue and discussion about the many issues pertaining to eating disorders. The ECED is an informal multidisciplinary network of people throughout Europe who work with eating disorder sufferers in a variety of contexts.

British Association for Counselling and Psychotherapy
BACP House, 35-37 Albert Street
Rugby, Warwickshire CV21 2SG, United Kingdom
Phone: 0870 443 5252
E-mail: bacp@bacp.co.uk
Website: www.bacp.co.uk

Provides lists of counselors in local areas.

Australia

Eating Disorders Foundation of New South Wales, Inc.
P.O. Box 532
Willoughby, NSW 2068, Australia
Phone: 9412 4499
Fax: 9413 4903
E-mail: edsn@edsn.asn.au
Website: www.edsn.asn.au

A nonprofit organization providing information about various eating disorders and services and resources to assist recovery, including support and information telephone line, support groups, newsletters and pamphlets, and training workshops.

Eating Disorders Foundation of Victoria Inc.
1513 High Street
Glen Iris, Victoria 3146, Australia
Phone: 9885 0318
Fax: 9885 1153
Website: www.eatingdisorders.org.au

A nonprofit organization that aims to support those affected by eating disorders and to better inform the community about disordered eating.

Anorexia and Bulimia Nervosa Association
1st Floor, Woodards House
47 Waymouth Street
Adelaide 5000, South Australia
Phone: 8212 1644
Fax: 8212 7991

Offers counseling, assistance, and support to families, partners, and friends. Promotes community awareness.

Eating Disorders Resource Centre
53 Railway Terrace
Milton, Queensland 4064, Australia
Phone: 3876 2500
Fax: 3511 6959
Website: www.uq.net.au/eda

A nonprofit providing information, support, and referral services for the state of Queensland, Australia.

Psychotherapy and Counseling Federation of Australia
P.O. Box 481
Carlton South, Victoria 3053, Australia
Phone: 9639 8330
Fax: 9639 8340
Website: www.pacfa.org.au/scripts/default.asp

This is an "umbrella" association composed of affiliated professional associations that represent various modalities within the disciplines of psychotherapy and counseling in the Australian community.

New Zealand

New Zealand Association of Counselors
3rd Floor, Federated Farmers Building
169 London Street
Hamilton 2015, New Zealand
Phone: 834 0220
E-mail: execofficer@nzac.org.nz
Fax: 834 0221
Website: www.nzac.org.nz

NZAC now represents approximately 2,500 counselors who work in education, health, justice, and social welfare government agencies, community-based social service agencies, Iwi Social Services, Pacific Island Organizations, private practice, and a range of ethnicity-specific helping agencies.

Eating Difficulties Education Network
4 Warnock Street
P.O. Box 78 005
Grey Lynn, Auckland, New Zealand
Phone: 378 9039
Fax: 378 9393

Eating Awareness Team
Caretaker's Cottage
Cramner Centre
Christchurch, New Zealand
Phone: 366 7725
Fax: 366 7720

International

International Eating Disorder Referral Organization
Website: www.edreferral.com

Provides information and treatment resources for all forms of eating disorders.

IAEDP—The International Association of Eating Disorders
    Professionals
P.O. Box 1295
Pekin, IL 61555-1295
Phone: (800) 800-8126
Fax: (309) 346-2874
Website: www.iaedp.com

Aims to provide a high level of professionalism among practitioners who treat those suffering from eating disorders by emphasizing ethical and professional standards, offering education and training in the field, and certifying those who have met professional requirements.

FURTHER READING

GENERAL

Agras, W. S., Eating Disorders, in A. F. Schatzberg and C. B. Nemeroff, Editors, *Textbook of Psychopharmacology*, 2003. Washington, DC: American Psychiatric Publishing Inc., pp. 1031–1040.

American Psychiatric Association, *Diagnostic and Statistical Manual of Mental Disorders*, Fourth Edition, Text Revision, 2000. Washington, DC: American Psychiatric Association.

American Psychiatric Association, Practice Guideline for the Treatment of Patients with Eating Disorders (Revision), *American Journal of Psychiatry*, 2000, *157* (Suppl.), pp. 1–39.

Cooper, Z., and C. G. Fairburn, The Eating Disorder Examination: A Semi-Structured Interview for the Assessment of the Specific Psychopathology of Eating Disorders. *International Journal of Eating Disorders*, 1987, *6*, 1–8.

Fairburn, C. G., and K. D. Brownell, Editors, *Eating Disorders and Obesity: A Comprehensive Handbook*, Second Edition, 2002. New York: Guilford Press.

Fairburn, C. G., and P. J. Harrison, Eating Disorders, *Lancet*, 2003, *361*, 407–416.

Fisher, M., M. Schneider, J. Burns, et al. Differences between Adolescents and Young Adults at Presentation to an Eating Disorder Program, *Journal of Adolescent Health*, 2001, *28*, 222–227.

Flament, M., S. Ledoux, P. Jeammet, et al., A Population Study of

Bulimia Nervosa and Subclinical Eating Disorders in Adolescence, in H. Steinhausen, Editor, *Eating Disorders in Adolescence: Anorexia and Bulimia Nervosa*, 1995, New York: Brunner/Mazel, pp. 21–36.

Gull, W., Anorexia Nervosa (Apepsia Hysterica, Anorexia Hysterica), *Transactions of the Clinical Society of London*, 1874, 7, 222–228.

Hoek, H., and D. van Hoeken, Review of Prevalence and Incidence of Eating Disorders, *International Journal of Eating Disorders*, 2003, *34*, 383–396.

Hsu, L. K., *Eating Disorders*, 1990. New York: Guilford Press.

Keys, A., J. Brozek, and A. Henschel, *The Biology of Human Starvation*, 1950. Minneapolis: University of Minnesota Press.

Lasegue, E., De l'Anorexie Hystérique, *Archives Générales de Médecine*, 1883, *21*, 384–403.

Lask, B., and R. Bryant-Waugh, Editors, *Anorexia Nervosa and Related Disorders in Childhood and Adolescence*, Second Edition, 2000. East Sussex, England: Psychology Press.

le Grange, D., and J. Lock, Bulimia Nervosa in Adolescents: Treatment, Eating Pathology, and Comorbidity. *South African Psychiatry Review*, 2002, *5*, 19–29.

le Grange, D., and J. Lock, The Dearth of Psychological Treatment Studies for Anorexia Nervosa. *International Journal of Eating Disorders*, in press.

Levenkron, S., *Anatomy of Anorexia*, 2001, New York: Norton.

Lucas, A. R., C. S. Crowson, W. M. O'Fallon, et al., The Ups and Downs of Anorexia Nervosa, *International Journal of Eating Disorders*, 1999, *26*, 397–405.

Natenshon, A. H., *When Your Child Has an Eating Disorder: A Step-by-Step Workbook for Parents and Other Caregivers*, 1999. San Francisco: Jossey-Bass.

Pirke, M., and P. Platte, Neurobiology of Eating Disorders in Adolescents, in H. Steinhausen, Editor, *Eating Disorders in Adolescence: Anorexia and Bulimia Nervosa*, 1995, New York: Brunner/Mazel, pp. 171–179.

Saraf, M., Holy Anorexia and Anorexia Nervosa: Society and Concept of Disease, *The Pharos*, 1998, *61*, 2–4.

Silverman, J., Charcot's Comments on the Therapeutic Role of Isolation in the Treatment of Anorexia Nervosa. *International Journal of Eating Disorders*, 1997, *21*, 295–298.

Smolack, L., M. Levine, and R. Striegel-Moore, *The Developmental Psychopathology of Eating Disorders*, 1996. Mahwah, NJ: Erlbaum.

Steiner, H., and J. Lock, Anorexia Nervosa and Bulimia Nervosa in Children and Adolescents: A Review of the Past 10 Years, *Journal of the American of Child and Adolescent Psychiatry*, 1998, *37*(4), 352–359.

Striegel-Moore, R. H., D. Leslie, S. A. Petrill, et al., One-Year Use and Cost of Inpatient and Outpatient Services among Female and Male Patients with an Eating Disorder: Evidence from a National Database of Health Insurance Claims, *International Journal of Eating Disorders*, 2000, *27*, 381–389.

Thompson, J. K., Editor, *Handbook of Eating Disorders and Obesity*, 2004. Hoboken, NJ: Wiley.

Treasure, J., *Anorexia Nervosa: A Survival Guide for Families, Friends, and Sufferers*, 1997. East Sussex, England: Psychology Press.

Vandereycken, W., Families of Patients with Eating Disorders, in C. G. Fairburn and K. Brownell, Editors, *Eating Disorders and Obesity: A Comprehensive Handbook*, Second Edition, 2002. New York: Guilford Press, pp. 215–220.

Wilson, G. T., and C. G. Fairburn, Treatments for Eating Disorders, in P. Nathan and J. Gorman, Editors, *A Guide to Treatments That Work*, 2002. New York: Oxford University Press, pp. 559–592.

RISKS FOR EATING DISORDERS

Agras, W. S., H. C. Kraemer, R. I. Berkowitz, et al., Does a Vigorous Feeding Style Influence Early Development of Adiposity?, *Journal of Pediatrics*, 1987, *110*(5), 799–804.

Attie, I., and J. Brooks-Gunn, Development of Eating Problems in Adolescent Girls: A Longitudinal Study. *Developmental Psychology*, 1989, *25*, 70–79.

Beren, S., H. A. Hayden, D. Wilfley, et al., Body-Dissatisfaction among Lesbian College Students: The Conflict of Straddling Mainstream and Lesbian Cultures, *Psychology of Women Quarterly*, 1997, *21*, 431–445.

Braun, D., S. R. Sunday, A. Huang, et al., More Males Seek Treatment for Eating Disorders, *International Journal of Eating Disorders*, 1999, *25*, 415–424.

Bravender, T., L. Roberston, E. R. Woods, et al., Is There an Increased Clinical Severity of Patients with Eating Disorders under Managed Care?, *Journal of Adolecent Health*, 1999, *24*, 422–426.

Bulik, C. M., Genetic and Biological Risk Factors, in J. K. Thompson, Editor, *Handbook of Eating Disorders and Obesity*, 2004. Hoboken, NJ: Wiley, pp. 3–16.

Bulik, C. M., J. Fear, and A. Pickering, Predictors of the Development of Bulimia Nervosa in Women with Anorexia Nervosa, *Journal of Nervous and Mental Disease*, 1997, *185*, 704–707.

Bulik, C. M., P. F. Sullivan, and K. S. Kendler, Heritability of Binge Eating and Broadly Defined Bulimia Nervosa, *Biological Psychiatry*, 1998, *44*, 1210–1218.

Carlat, D. J., C. A. Camargo, Jr., and D. B. Herzog, Eating Disorders in Males: A Report on 135 Patients, *American Journal of Psychiatry*, 1997, *154*(8), 1127–1132.

Casper, R., and M. Troiani, Family Functioning in Anorexia by Subtype, *International Journal of Eating Disorders*, 2001, *30*, 338–342.

Davis, C., and M. Katzman, Perfectionism as Acculturation: Psychological Correlates of Eating Problems in Chinese Male and Female Students Living in the United States, *International Journal of Eating Disorders*, 1999, *25*, 65–70.

Drucker, R. R., L. D. Hammer, W. S. Agras, et al., Can Mothers Influence Their Child's Eating Behavior?, *Journal of Developmental and Behavioral Pediatrics*, 1999, *20*(2), 88–92.

Fairburn, C. G., Z. Cooper, H. A. Doll, et al., Risk Factors for Anorexia Nervosa: Three Integrated Case–Control Comparisons, *Archives of General Psychiatry*, 1999, *56*, 468–476.

Fairburn, C. G., P. J. Cowen, and P. J. Harrison, Twin Studies and the Etiology of Eating Disorders, *International Journal of Eating Disorders*, 1999, *26*, 349–358.

Fairburn, C. G., H. A. Doll, S. L. Welch, et al., Risk Factors for Binge Eating Disorder: A Community-Based, Case–Control Study, *Archives of General Psychiatry*, 1998, *55*(5), 425–432.

Fairburn, C. G., S. L. Welch, H. A. Doll, et al., Risk Factors for Bulimia Nervosa: A Community-Based Case–Control Study, *Archives of General Psychiatry*, 1997, *54*(6), 509–517.

Field, A., Risk Factors for Eating Disorders: An Evaluation of the Evidence, in J. K. Thompson, Editor, *Handbook of Eating Disorders and Obesity*, 2004. Hoboken, NJ: Wiley, pp. 17–32.

Fouts, G., and K. Burggraf, Television Situation Comedies: Female Body Images and Verbal Reinforcements, *Sex Roles*, 1999, *40*, 473–481.

Frank, G., W. H. Kaye, C. C. Meltzer, et al., Reduced 5-HT2A Receptor Binding after Recovery from Anorexia Nervosa, *Biological Psychiatry*, 2002, *52*, 896–906.

Franko, D., and M. Omori, Subclinical Eating Disorders in Adolescent Women: A Test of the Continuity Hypothesis and Its Psychological Correlates, *Journal of Adolescence*, 1999, *22*, 389–398.

French, S. A., N. Leffert, M. Story, et al., Adolescent Binge/Purge and

Weight Loss Behaviors: Associations with Developmental Assets, *Journal of Adolescent Health*, 2001, *28*, 211–221.

Gowen, L., C. Hayward, J. D. Killen, et al., Acculturation and Eating Disorder Symptoms in Adolescent Girls, *Journal of Research on Adolescence*, 1999, *9*, 67–83.

Gunewardene, A., G. Huon, and R. Zheng, Exposure to Westernization and Dieting: A Cross-Cultural Study, *International Journal of Eating Disorders*, 2001, *29*, 289–293.

Hill, A., and R. Bhatti, Body Shape Perception and Dieting in Pre-Adolescent British Asian Girls: Links with Eating Disorders, *International Journal of Eating Disorders*, 1995, *17*, 175–183.

Humphrey, L., Structural Analysis of Parent–Child Relationships in Eating Disorders, *Journal of Abnormal Psychology*, 1986, *95*, 395–402.

Humphrey, L., Comparison of Bulimic–Anorexic and Nondistressed Families Using Structural Analysis of Behavior, *Journal of the American Academy of Child and Adolescent Psychiatry*, 1987, *26*, 248–255.

Killen, J. D., C. B. Taylor, and C. Hayward, Weight Concerns Influence the Development of Eating Disorders, *Journal of Consulting and Clinical Psychology*, 1996, *64*, 936–940.

Killen, J. D., C. B. Taylor, M. J. Telch, et al., Self-Induced Vomiting and Laxative Use among Teenagers: Precursors of the Binge–Purge Syndrome?, *Journal of the American Medical Association*, 1986, *255*, 1447–1449.

Lake, A., P. Staiger, and H. Glowinski, Effects of Western Culture on Women's Attitudes to Eating and Perceptions of Body Shape, *International Journal of Eating Disorders*, 2000, *27*, 83–89.

Lee, S., Self-Starvation in Context: Towards a Culturally Sensitive Understanding of Anorexia Nervosa, *Social Science and Medicine*, 1995, *41*, 25–36.

Levine, M., and K. Harrison, Media's Role in the Perpetuation and Prevention of Negative Body Image and Disordered Eating, in J. K. Thompson, Editor, *Handbook of Eating Disorders and Obesity*, 2004. Hoboken, NJ: Wiley, pp. 695–717.

Marchi, M., and P. Cohen, Early Childhood Eating Behaviors and Adolescent Eating Disorders, *Journal of the American Academy of Child and Adolescent Psychiatry*, 1990, *29*, 112–117.

McClelland, L., and A. H. Crisp, Anorexia Nervosa and Social Class, *International Journal of Eating Disorders*, 2001, *29*, 150–156.

Patton, G. C., R. Selzer, C. Coffey, et al., Onset of Adolescent Eating Disorders: Population Based Cohort Study over 3 Years, *British Medical Journal*, 1999, *318*, 765–768.

Pope, H. G., R. Olivardia, A. Gruber, et al., Evolving Ideals of Male Body Image as Seen through Action Toys, *International Journal of Eating Disorders*, 1999, *26*, 65–72.

Steiner, H., W. Kwan, T. G. Schaffer, et al., Risk and Protective Factors for Juvenile Eating Disorders, *European Child and Adolescent Psychiatry*, 2003, *12*(Suppl. 1), 38–46.

Stice, E., and W. S. Agras, Predicting Onset and Cessation of Bulimic Behaviors during Adolescence, *Behavior Therapy*, 1998, *29*, 257–276.

Strober, M., R. Freeman, C. Lampert, et al., Controlled Family Study of Anorexia Nervosa and Bulimia Nervosa: Evidence of Shared Liability and Transmission of Partial Syndromes, *American Journal of Psychiatry*, 2000, *157*, 393–401.

Strober, M., and L. Humphrey, Family Contributions to the Etiology and Course of Anorexia and Bulimia, *Journal of Clinical Psychology*, 1987, *55*, 654–659.

Welch, S. L., H. A. Doll, and C. G. Fairburn, Life Events and the Onset of Bulimia Nervosa: A Controlled Study, *Psychological Medicine*, 1997, *27*(3), 515–522.

Welch, S. L., and C. G. Fairburn, Childhood Sexual and Physical Abuse as Risk Factors for the Development of Bulimia Nervosa: A Community-Based Case Control Study [See Comments], *Child Abuse and Neglect*, 1996, *20*(7), 633–642.

Welch, S. L., and C. G. Fairburn, Sexual Abuse and Bulimia Nervosa: Three Integrated Case Control Comparisons, *American Journal of Psychiatry*, 1994, *151*(3), 402–407.

Whelan, E., and P. J. Cooper, The Association between Childhood Feeding Problems and Maternal Eating Disorder: A Community Study, *Psychological Medicine*, 2000, *30*, 69–77.

Wonderlich, S. A., R. D. Crosby, J. E. Mitchell, et al., Eating Disturbance and Sexual Trauma in Childhood and Adulthood, *International Journal of Eating Disorders*, 2001, *30*, 401–412.

Woodside, D. B., C. M. Bulik, K. A. Halmi, et al., Personality, Perfectionism, and Attitudes toward Eating in Parents of Individuals with Eating Disorders, *International Journal of Eating Disorders*, 2002, *31*, 290–299.

MEDICAL PROBLEMS ASSOCIATED WITH EATING DISORDERS

American Academy of Pediatrics, Policy Statement: Identifying and Treating Eating Disorders, *Pediatrics*, 2003, *111*, 204–211.

Fisher, M., N. H. Golden, D. K. Katzman, et al., Eating Disorders in Adolescents: A Background Paper, *Journal of Adolescent Health*, 1995, *16*, 420–437.

Garfinkel, P., E. Lin, and P. Goering, Should Amenorrhoea Be Necessary for the Diagnosis of Anorexia Nervosa?: Evidence from a Canadian Community Sample, *British Journal of Psychiatry*, 1996, *168*, 500–506.

Golden, N. H., D. K. Katzman, R. E Kreipe, et al., Eating Disorders in Adolescents: Position Paper of the Society for Adolescent Medicine, *Journal of Adolescent Health*, 2003, *33*, 496–503.

Herzog, D. B., D. N. Greenwood, D. J. Dorer, et al., Mortality in Eating Disorders: A Descriptive Study, *International Journal of Eating Disorders*, 2000, *28*, 20–26.

Lock, J., B. Reisel, and H. Steiner, Associated Health Risks of Adolescents with Disordered Eating: How Different Are They from Their Peers?: Results from a High School Survey, *Child Psychiatry and Human Development*, 2001, *31*, 249–265.

Mitchell, J., H. C. Seim, and E. Colon, Medical Complications and Medical Management of Bulimia, *Annals of Internal Medicine*, 1987, *107*, 71–77.

Patton, G. C., Mortality in Eating Disorders, *Psychological Medicine*, 1988, *18*, 947–951.

Rome, E., and S. Ammerman, Medical Complications of Eating Disorders: An Update, *Journal of Adolecent Health*, 2003, *33*, 418–426.

Society of Adolescent Medicine, Eating Disorders in Adolescents: Position Paper of the Society for Adolescent Medicine, *Journal of Adolecent Health*, 2003, *33*, 496–503.

Steiger, H., L. Gauvin, M. Israel, et al., Association of Serotonin and Cortisol Indices with Childhood Abuse in Bulimia Nervosa, *Archives of General of Psychiatry*, 2001, *58*, 837–843.

Sullivan, P. F., Mortality in Anorexia Nervosa, *American Journal of Psychiatry*, 1995, *152*, 1073–1074.

Swenne, I., Heart Risk Associated with Weight Loss in Anorexia Nervosa and Eating Disorders: Electrocardiographic Changes during the Early Phase of Refeeding, *Acta Pediatrica*, 2000, *89*, 447–452.

PSYCHOLOGICAL TREATMENTS FOR EATING DISORDERS

Agras, W. S., and R. F. Apple, *Overcoming Eating Disorders: A Cognitive-Behavioral Treatment for Bulimia Nervosa and Binge Eating Disorder:*

Therapist Guide, 1997. San Antonio, TX: Psychological Corporation.

Agras, W. S., T. Walsh, C. G. Fairburn, et al., A Multicenter Comparison of Cognitive-Behavioral Therapy and Interpersonal Psychotherapy for Bulimia Nervosa, *Archives of General Psychiatry*, 2000, *57*, 459–466.

Apple, R. F., and W. S. Agras, *Overcoming Eating Disorders: A Cognitive-Behavioral Treatment for Bulimia Nervosa and Binge Eating Disorder: Client Workbook*, 1997. San Antonio, TX: Psychological Corporation.

Bowers, W. A., K. Evans, D. le Grange, et al., Treatment of Adolescent Eating Disorders, in M. Reinecke, F. Dattilio, and A. Freeman, Editors, *Cognitive Therapy with Children and Adolescents: A Casebook for Clinical Practice*, Second Edition, 2003. New York: Guilford Press, pp. 247–280.

Bruch, H., *Eating Disorders: Obesity, Anorexia Nervosa, and the Person Within*, 1973. New York: Basic Books.

Bruch, H., *The Golden Cage: The Enigma of Anorexia Nervosa*, 1978. Cambridge, MA: Harvard University Press.

Channon, S., P. de Silva, D. Hemsley, et al., A Controlled Trial of Cognitive-Behavioural and Behavioural Treatment of Anorexia Nervosa, *Behaviour Research and Therapy*, 1989, *27*(5), 529–535.

Cooper, P. J., and J. Steere, A Comparison of Two Psychological Treatments for Bulimia Nervosa: Implications for Models of Maintenance, *Behaviour Research and Therapy*, 1995, *33*, 875–885.

Crisp, A. H., *Anorexia Nervosa: Let Me Be*, 1980. London: Academic Press.

Crisp, A. H., Anorexia Nervosa as Flight from Growth: Assessment and Treatment Based on the Model, in D. M. Garner and P. E. Garfinkel, Editors, *Handbook of Treatment for Eating Disorders*, Second Edition, 1997. New York: Guilford Press, pp. 248–277.

Crisp, A. H., K. Norton, S. Gowers, et al., A Controlled Study of the Effect of Therapies Aimed at Adolescent and Family Psychopathology in Anorexia Nervosa, *British Journal of Psychiatry*, 1991, *159*, 325–333.

Dare, C., and I. Eisler, Family Therapy for Anorexia Nervosa, in I. Cooper and A. Stein, Editors, *The Nature and Management of Feeding Problems in Young People*, 1992. New York: Harwood Academics.

Dare, C., and I. Eisler, Family Therapy for Anorexia Nervosa, in D. M. Garner and P. Garfinkel, Editors, *Handbook of Treatment for Eating Disorders*, Second Edition, 1997. New York: Guilford Press, pp. 307–324.

Dare, C., and I. Eisler, A Multi-Family Group Day Treatment Programme for Adolescent Eating Disorders, *European Eating Disorders Review*, 2000, *8*, 4–18.

Dare, C., I. Eisler, G. Russell, et al., Psychological Therapies for Adults with Anorexia Nervosa: Randomised Controlled Trial of Outpatient Treatments, *British Journal of Psychiatry*, 2001, *178*, 216–221.

Dodge, E., M. Hodes, I. Eisler, et al., Family Therapy for Bulimia Nervosa in Adolescents: An Exploratory Study, *Journal of Family Therapy*, 1995, *17*, 59–77.

Eisler, I., C. Dare, M. Hodes, et al., Family Therapy for Adolescent Anorexia Nervosa: The Results of a Controlled Comparison of Two Family Interventions, *Journal of Child Psychology and Psychiatry*, 2000, *41*(6), 727–736.

Eisler, I., C. Dare, G. F. Russell, et al., Family and Individual Therapy in Anorexia Nervosa: A Five-Year Follow-Up, *Archives of General Psychiatry*, 1997, *54*, 1025–1030.

Fairburn, C., A Cognitive Behavioral Approach to the Treatment of Bulimia, *Psychological Medicine*, 1981, *11*(4), 707–711.

Fairburn, C. G., Eating Disorders, in D. Clark and C. G. Fairburn, Editors, *Cognitive-Behavioral Therapy: Science and Practice*, 1997. Oxford, England: Oxford University Press, pp. 160–192.

Fairburn, C. G., Interpersonal Psychotherapy for Bulimia Nervosa, in D. M. Garner and P. E. Garfinkel, Editors, *Handbook of Treatment for Eating Disorders*, Second Edition, 1997. New York: Guilford Press, pp. 278–294.

Fairburn, C. G., *Overcoming Binge Eating*, 1995. New York: Guilford Press.

Fairburn, C. G., R. Jones, R. C. Peveler, et al., Three Psychological Treatments for Bulimia Nervosa: A Comparative Trial, *Archives of General Psychiatry*, 1991, *48*(5), 463–469.

Fairburn, C. G., J. Kirk, M. O'Connor, et al., A Comparison of Two Psychological Treatments for Bulimia Nervosa, *Behaviour Research and Therapy*, 1986, *24*(6), 629–643.

Fairburn, C. G., R. Shafran, and Z. Cooper, A Cognitive Behavioural Theory of Anorexia Nervosa, *Behaviour Research and Therapy*, 1999, *37*(1), 1–13.

Haley, J., *Uncommon Therapy: The Psychiatric Techniques of Milton H. Erickson*, 1973. New York: Norton.

Hall, A., and A. H. Crisp, Brief Psychotherapy in the Treatment of Anorexia Nervosa: Outcome at One Year, *British Journal of Psychiatry*, 1987, *151*, 185–191.

Krautter, T., and J. Lock, Is Manualized Family-Based Treatment for

Adolescent Anorexia Nervosa Acceptable to Patients?: Patient Satisfaction at End of Treatment, *Journal of Family Therapy*, 2004, *26*, 65–81.

le Grange, D., I. Eisler, C. Dare, et al., Evaluation of Family Treatments in Adolescent Anorexia Nervosa: A Pilot Study, *International Journal of Eating Disorders*, 1992, *12*(4), 347–357.

le Grange, D., and T. Gelman, The Patient's Perspective of Treatment in Eating Disorders: A Preliminary Study, *South African Journal of Psychology*, 1998, *28*, 182–186.

le Grange, D., J. Lock, and M. Dymek, Family-Based Therapy for Adolescents with Bulimia Nervosa, *American Journal of Psychotherapy*, 2003, *67*, 237–251.

Lemmon, C., and A. Josephson, Family Therapy for Eating Disorders, *Psychiatric Clinics of North America*, 2001, *10*, 519–542.

Liebman, R., J. Sargent, and M. Silver, A Family Systems Approach to the Treatment of Anorexia Nervosa, *Journal of the American Academy of Child and Adolescent Psychiatry*, 1983, *22*, 128–133.

Lock, J., Treating Adolescents with Eating Disorders in the Family Context: Empirical and Theoretical Considerations, *Child and Adolescent Psychiatric Clinics of North America*, 2002, *11*, 331–342.

Lock, J., What Is the Best Way to Treat Adolescents with Anorexia Nervosa?, *Eating Disorders*, 2001, *9*, 299–302.

Lock, J., and D. le Grange, Can Family-Based Treatment of Anorexia Nervosa Be Manualized?, *Journal of Psychotherapy Practice and Research*, 2001, *10*, 253–261.

Lock, J., D. le Grange, W. S. Agras, et al., *Treatment Manual for Anorexia Nervosa: A Family-Based Approach*, 2001. New York: Guilford Press.

Madanes, C., *Strategic Family Therapy*, 1981. San Francisco: Jossey-Bass.

Minuchin, S., B. Rosman, and I. Baker, *Psychosomatic Families: Anorexia Nervosa in Context*, 1978. Cambridge, MA: Harvard University Press.

Palazzoli, M., *Self-Starvation: From the Intrapsychic to the Transpersonal Approach to Anorexia Nervosa*, 1974. London: Chaucer.

Pike, K. M., B. T. Walsh, K. Vitousek, et al., Cognitive Behavior Therapy in the Posthospitalization Treatment of Anorexia Nervosa, *American Journal of Psychiatry*, 2004, *160*, 2046–2049.

Robin, A. L., P. T. Siegel, A. W. Moye, et al., A Controlled Comparison of Family versus Individual Therapy for Adolescents with Anorexia Nervosa, *Journal of the American Academy of Child and Adolescent Psychiatry*, 1999, *38*(12), 1482–1489.

Russell, G. F., G. I. Szmukler, C. Dare, et al., An Evaluation of Family

Therapy in Anorexia Nervosa and Bulimia Nervosa, *Archives of General Psychiatry*, 1987, *44*(12), 1047–1056.

Safer, D. L., C. Telch, F., and W. S. Agras, Dialectical Behavior Therapy for Bulimia Nervosa, *American Journal of Psychiatry*, 2001, *158*, 632–634.

Scholz, M., and K. E. Asen, Multiple Family Therapy with Eating Disordered Adolescents, *European Eating Disorders Review*, 2001, *9*, 33–42.

Schwartz, R., M. Barrett, and G. Saba, Family Therapy for Bulimia, in D. M. Garner and P. E. Garfinkel, Editors, *Handbook of Psychotherapy for Anorexia Nervosa and Bulimia*, 1985. New York: Guilford Press, pp. 280–310.

Stewart, A., Disorders of Eating Control in Adolescents, in P. Graham, Editor, *Cognitive-Behavioral Treatment with Children and Adolescents*, Cambridge: Cambridge University Press, in press.

Stierlin, H., and G. Weber, *Unlocking the Family Door: A Systemic Approach to the Understanding and Treatment of Anorexia Nervosa*, 1989. New York: Brunner/Mazel.

Treasure, J., G. Todd, M. Brolly, et al., A Pilot Study of a Randomised Trial of Cognitive Analytical Therapy vs. Educational Behavioral Therapy for Adult Anorexia Nervosa, *Behaviour Research and Therapy*, 1995, *33*, 363–367.

Vitousek, K., S. Watson, and G. T. Wilson, Enhancing Motivation for Change in Treatment-Resistant Eating Disorders, *Clinical Psychology Review*, 1998, *18*(4), 391–420.

White, M., and D. Epston, *Narrative Means to Therapeutic Ends*, 1990. New York: Norton.

Whittal, M. L., W. S. Agras, and R. A. Gould, Bulimia Nervosa: A Meta-Analysis of Psychosocial and Pharmacological Treatments, *Behavior Therapy*, 1999, *30*, 117–135.

Wilson, G. T., C. G. Fairburn, W. S. Agras, et al., Cognitive Behavioral Therapy for Bulimia Nervosa: Time Course and Mechanisms of Change, *Journal of Consulting and Clinical Psychology*, 2002, *70*, 267–274.

PHARMACOLOGICAL TREATMENTS
FOR EATING DISORDERS

Attia, E., C. Haiman, B. T. Walsh, et al., Does Fluoxetine Augment the Inpatient Treatment of Anorexia Nervosa?, *American Journal of Psychiatry*, 1998, *155*(4), 548–551.

Attia, E., L. Mayer, and E. Killory, Medication Response in the Treatment of Patients with Anorexia Nervosa, *Journal of Psychiatric Practice*, 2001, 7, 157–162.

Fluoexetine Bulimia Nervosa Group, Fluoxetine in the Treatment of Bulimia Nervosa, *Archives of General Psychiatry*, 1992, 49, 139–147.

Halmi, C. A., E. D. Eckert, and T. J. Ladu, Treatment Efficacy of Cyproheptadine and Amitryptiline, *Archives of General Psychiatry*, 1986, 43, 177–181.

Kaye, W. H., An Open Trial of Fluoxetine in Patients with Anorexia Nervosa, *Journal of Clinical Psychiatry*, 1991, 52, 464–471.

Kaye, W. H., K. Grendall, and M. Strober, Serotonin Neuronal Function and Selective Serotonin Reuptake Inhibitor Treatment in Anorexia Nervosa, *Biological Psychiatry*, 1998, 44, 825–838.

Kaye, W. H., T. Nagata, T. E. Weltzin, et al., Double-Blind Placebo-Controlled Administration of Fluoxetine in Restricting and Restricting–Purging Type Anorexia Nervosa, *Biological Psychiatry*, 2001, 49, 644–652.

Malina, A., J. Gaskill, C. McConaha, et al., Olanzapine Treatment of Anorexia Nervosa: A Retrospective Study, *International Journal of Eating Disorders*, 2003, 33, 234–237.

Walsh, B. T., G. T. Wilson, K. L. Loeb, et al., Medication and Psychotherapy in the Treatment of Bulimia Nervosa, *American Journal of Psychiatry*, 1997, 154(4), 523–531.

COMORBID PSYCHIATRIC PROBLEMS WITH EATING DISORDERS

Casper, R., D. Hedeker, and J. McClough, Personality Dimensions in Eating Disorders and Their Relevance for Subtyping, *Journal of the American Academy of Child and Adolescent Psychiatry*, 1992, 31, 830–840.

Godart, N. T., M. F. Flament, Y. Lecrubier, et al., Anxiety Disorders in Anorexia Nervosa and Bulimia Nervosa: Comorbidity and Chronology of Appearance, *European Psychiatry*, 2000, 15, 38–45.

Godart, N., M. F. Flament, F. Perdereau, et al., Comorbidity between Eating Disorders and Anxiety Disorders: A Review, *International Journal of Eating Disorders*, 2002, 32, 253–270.

Herzog, D. B., M. B. Keller, N. R. Sacks, et al., Psychiatric Comorbidity in Treatment-Seeking Anorexics and Bulimics, *Journal of the American Academy of Child and Adolescent Psychiatry*, 1992, 31(5), 810–818.

Herzog, D. B., K. M. Nussbaum, and A. K. Marmor, Comorbidity and

Outcome in Eating Disorders, *Psychiatric Clinics of North America*, 1996, *19*(4), 843–859.

Klump, K., C. M. Bulik, C. Pollice, et al., Temperament and Character in Women with Anorexia Nervosa, *Journal of Nervous and Mental Diseases*, 2000, *188*, 559–567.

Telch, C. F., and E. Stice, Psychiatric Comorbidity in Women with Binge Eating Disorder: Prevalence Rates from a Non-Treatment-Seeking Sample, *Journal of Consulting and Clinical Psychology*, 1998, *66*(5), 768–776.

Vitousek, K., and F. Manke, Personality Variables and Disorders in Anorexia Nervosa and Bulimia Nervosa, *Journal of Abnormal Psychology*, 1994, *103*, 137–147.

Wonderlich, S., Personality and Eating Disorders, in C. G. Fairburn and K. Brownell, Editors, *Eating Disorders and Obesity: A Comprehensive Handbook*, Second Edition, 2002. New York: Guilford Press, pp. 204–209.

RECOVERY FROM AND OUTCOME OF EATING DISORDERS

Agras, W. S., S. J. Crow, K. A. Halmi, et al., Outcome Predictors for the Cognitive Behavioral Treatment of Bulimia Nervosa: Data from a Multisite Study, *American Journal of Psychiatry*, 2000, *157*, 1302–1308.

Bryant-Waugh, R., J. Knibbs, A. Fosson, et al., Long-Term Follow-Up of Patients with Early Onset Anorexia Nervosa, *Archives of Diseases of Childhood*, 1988, *63*, 5–9.

Cachelin, F. M., R. H. Striegel-Moore, K. A. Elder, et al., Natural Course of a Community Sample of Women with Binge Eating Disorder, *International Journal of Eating Disorders*, 1999, *25*(1), 45–54.

Collings, S., and M. King, Ten-Year Follow-Up of 50 Patients with Bulimia Nervosa, *British Journal of Psychiatry*, 1994, *164*, 80–87.

Deter, J., and W. Herzog, Anorexia Nervosa in a Long-Term Perspective: Results of the Heidelberg–Mannheim Study, *Psychosomatic Medicine*, 1994, *56*, 20–27.

Deter, J., W. Herzog, and E. Petzold, The Heidelberg–Mannheim Study: Long-Term Follow-Up of Anorexia Nervosa Patients at the University Medical Center—Background and Preliminary Results, in W. Herzog and W. Vandereycken, Editors, *The Course of Eating Disorders*, 1992. Berlin: Springer-Verlag, pp. 71–84.

Eckert, E. D., K. A. Halmi, P. Marchi, et al., Ten-Year Follow-Up of Anorexia Nervosa: Clinical Course and Outcome, *Psychological Medicine*, 1995, *25*, 143–156.

Eddy, K., P. K. Keel, D. J. Dorer, et al., Longitundinal Comparison of Anorexia Nervosa Subtypes, *International Journal of Eating Disorders*, 2002, *31*, 191–202.

Engel, K., A. E. Meyer, M. Henze, et al., Long-Term Outcome in Anorexia Nervosa Inpatients, in W. Herzog and W. Vandereycken, Editors, *The Course of Eating Disorders*, 1992. Berlin: Springer-Verlag, pp. 167–181.

Fairburn, C. G., Z. Cooper, H. A. Doll, et al., The Natural Course of Bulimia Nervosa and Binge Eating Disorder in Young Women, *Archives of General Psychiary*, 2000, *57*, 659–665.

George, D., S. R. Weiss, H. E. Gwirtzman, et al., Anorexia Nervosa: A 25 Year Retrospective Study from 1958–1982, *International Journal of Eating Disorders*, 1987, *6*, 321–330.

Gillberg, I., M. Rastam, and L. Gillberg, Anorexia Nerovsa Outcome: Six-Year Controlled Longitudinal Study of 51 Cases Including a Population Cohort, *Journal of the American Academy of Child and Adolescent Psychiatry*, 1994, *33*, 729–739.

Hawley, R., The Outcome of Anorexia Nervosa in Younger Subjects, *British Journal of Psychiatry*, 1985, *146*, 657–660.

Herzog, D. B., D. J. Dorer, P. K. Keel, et al., Recovery and Relapse in Anorexia and Bulimia Nervosa: A 7.5-Year Follow-Up Study, *Journal of the American Academy of Child and Adolescent Psychiatry*, 1999, *38*(7), 829–837.

Jenkins, M., An Outcome Study of Anorexia Nervosa in an Adolescent Unit, *Journal of Adolescence*, 1987, *10*, 71–81.

Jones, L., Long-Term Outcome of Anorexia Nervosa, *Behavioral Change*, 1993, *10*, 835–842.

Kaye, W. H., C. G. Greeno, H. Moss, et al., Alterations in Serotonin Activity and Psychiatric Symptoms after Recovery from Bulimia Nervosa, *Archives of General Psychiatry*, 1998, *55*, 927–935.

Keel, P. K., J. E. Mitchell, K. B. Miller, et al., Long-Term Outcome of Bulimia Nervosa, *Archives of General Psychiatry*, 1999, *56*(1), 63–69.

Keel, P. K., J. E. Mitchell, K. B. Miller, et al., Social Adjustment over 10 Years Following Diagnosis with Bulimia Nervosa, *International Journal of Eating Disorders*, 2000, *27*(1), 21–28.

Olmsted, M. P., A. S. Kaplan, and W. Rockert, Rate and Prediction of Relapse in Bulimia Nervosa, *American Journal of Psychiatry*, 1994, *151*, 738–743.

Srinivasagam, N. M., W. H. Kaye, K. H. Plotnicov, et al., Persistent Perfectionism, Symmetry, and Exactness after Long-Term Recovery from Anorexia Nervosa, *American Journal of Psychiatry*, 1995, *152*, 1630–1634.

Steinhausen, H., C. Rauss-Mason, and R. Seidel, Short-Term and Intermediate-Term Outcome in Adolescent Eating Disorders, *Acta Psychiatrica Scandinavica*, 1993, *88*, 169–173.

Zipfel, S., B. Lowe, D. L. Reas, et al., Long-Term Prognosis in Anorexia Nervosa: Lessons from a 21-Year Follow-Up Study, *Lancet*, 2000, *355*, 721–722.

INDEX